The
TV Watcher's
Workout

Did you know . . .

that over 97 million
Americans are
overweight
or out of shape?

I couldn't believe it
either.

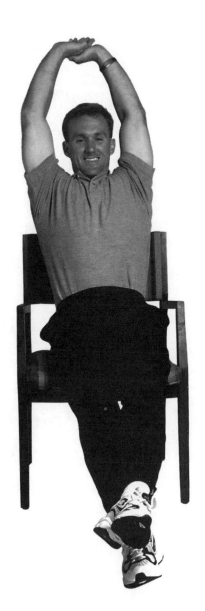

"Maybe," I thought,
"if those 97 million people didn't
have to change their lifestyle . . .

. . . didn't have to give up
too much time . . .

. . . could even exercise
in front of the TV! . . .

maybe, just then,
I'd be able to help some of those
people get back in shape."

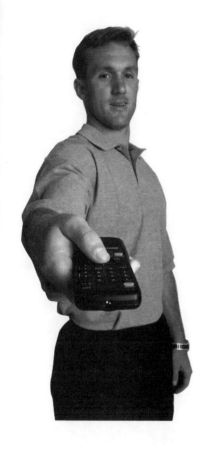

I'm Stew Smith,

a former
US Navy SEAL,

and this is . . .

The
TV Watcher's
Workout!

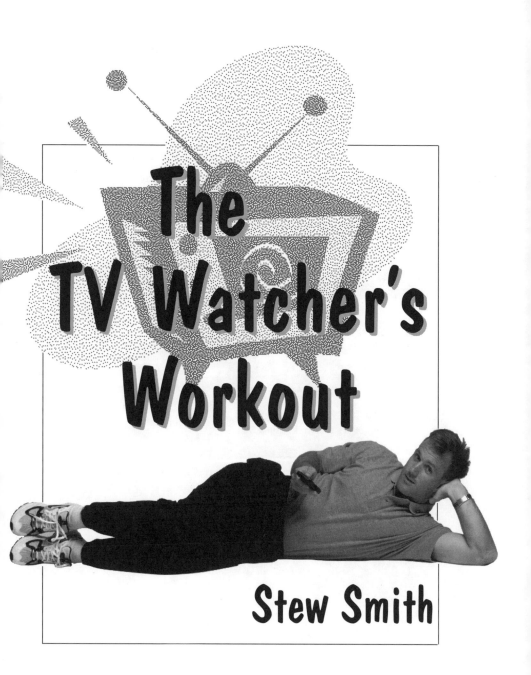

The TV Watcher's Workout

Stew Smith

FIVE STAR FITNESS
New York

Five Star Fitness
An Independent Imprint of Hatherleigh Press

Copyright © 1999 by Stewart Smith

Five Star Fitness
An Independent Imprint of Hatherleigh Press
1114 First Avenue, Suite 500
New York, NY 10021
1-800-906-1234
www.getfitnow.com

Before beginning any strenuous exercise program consult your physician. The author and publisher of this book and workout disclaim any liability, personal or professional, resulting from the misapplication of any of the training procedures described in this publication.

All Five Star Fitness titles are available for bulk purchase, special promotions, and premiums. For more information, please contact the manager of our Special Sales department at 1-800-906-1234.

Library of Congress Cataloging in-Publication Data

Smith, Stew, 1969–
  The TV watcher's workout / Stew Smith.
     p.   cm.
  ISBN 1-57826-020-5 (alk. paper)
  1. Exercise.   2. Television viewers—Health and hygiene.
  I. Title.
  RA781.S617   1999
  613.7'1—cc21   98-40697
                                                                          CIP

Cover design by Gary Szczecina
Text design and composition by John Reinhardt Book Design
Photographed by Peter Field Peck with Canon® cameras and lenses on Fuji®
print and slide film

Printed in Canada on acid-free paper

10   9   8   7   6   5   4   3   2

Dedication

This workout program is dedicated to my parents, who work all day at their own business, come home, eat a big dinner, watch a few television programs, and fall asleep. This is not unlike the daily routine of millions of Americans who spend more time making money than they do enjoying it.

I had asked my parents to exercise with me for years and nothing worked. Nothing motivated them! I even tried the guilt technique (you know, the one our parents used on all of us growing up). I even tried to scare them! I would ask, "Why are you working so hard to save for your retirement when you may not even be healthy enough to enjoy it?" This opened their eyes a bit. But they would only use a workout that didn't take a lot of time, require working out in public, or buying any fancy equipment. I was willing to compromise, and the *TV Watcher's Workout* was born!

My motto became: "Don't change your lifestyle to fit your workout, change your workout to fit your lifestyle."

Well, this appealed to my parents, who had to spend only minutes a day stretching, performing basic calisthenics, light resistance training, and walking in order to get in shape. Now, they have the confidence and ability to move to the next level of fitness. They are presently walking several miles a week and increasing the repetitions on the exercises.

I wrote this book for my parents and other people like them. I want my infant daughter to grow up with healthy grandparents. Plus, I personally feel that this workout will help you on your journey to healthy living. I hope you use this workout for several months and keep moving onto more challenging exercise programs when you have finished this program. Look for our *Five Star Fitness Series* for help with the next level of fitness . . .

Good Luck!

Acknowledgments

First let me thank the wonderful staff of **Hatherleigh Press** and **Five Star Fitness**. You have all been both professional and dedicated to producing excellent work.

Special thanks to **Andrew Flach**, who saw the potential of this book when other publishers did not.

Thanks also to **Susan Ruszala**, who added so much creativity to the *TV Watcher's Workout* and **Peter Peck**, whose mastery of the camera can make even me look okay . . . Thanks to you all, and I look forward to working with you in the future.

Special thanks also to **Rockefeller University Press**, who kindly provided us with our "armchair," and to **Dom's Deli**, who filled our fridge with their delicious food.

Contents

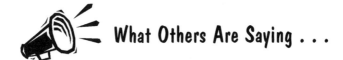 **What Others Are Saying . . .**

Our son Stewart has been a workout fanatic since he was thirteen years old. One day, he realized that we (his parents) were not! Well, ever since that day, Stewart has tried to motivate us to begin an exercise program. About all we ever did was walk around the neighborhood once in a while. When he went away to the Naval Academy, he continued to harass us to get out and exercise. Honestly, we were working long hours, coming home hungry and exhausted, watching a little TV, and going to bed.

Wouldn't you know it, he came up with a workout that fit into that schedule. And believe it or not, drinking more water, stretching and doing a few repetitions of the exercises really has worked. It has been over five years since Stewart introduced us to this program and we are actually healthier, lighter, and have more energy than we did in our twenties. It works—give it a try!

Jim and Rae Smith

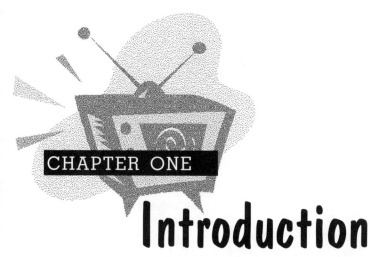

CHAPTER ONE

Introduction

There is no magic pill for weight loss and healthy living. The only true cure is eating right and getting up off the couch to exercise. It does not take several hours a day to become physically fit —only minutes a day will help you become healthier and have more energy than you have had in years.

Recently, the National Institute of Health (NIH) announced the results of a national study on the weight and body fat standards of Americans. The study was shocking because it revealed that approximately 97 million Americans, or over 40% of our population, are overweight. This statistic is extremely alarming, because you CANNOT be healthy and overweight. The two just do not mix.

Many Americans today spend most of their time trying to make money and less time being able to enjoy it. The problem with this mentality will be evident in later years, when those same Americans can't enjoy their retirement because of clogged arteries, strokes, arthritis, and other degenerative diseases caused by inactivity. All of which can be prevented or delayed by exercising—now.

It has been proven over and over again that regular physical activity is effective in increasing your energy level, resistance to illness, and self-esteem. With a good diet, a regular workout program promotes good health by reducing the chance of heart disease, obesity, and some forms of cancer, and lowers the risk of high blood pressure. Working out and maintaining a healthy lifestyle will make you feel better about yourself, without a doubt. The immediate and long-term benefits of beginning a fitness program, no matter how basic, are easily evident:

Immediate	Long Term
• increased energy level	• longer, healthier life
• stress reliever	• fewer illnesses (plus less medical expenses!)
• increased metabolism	• increased flexibility of the joints
• calorie burner	• weight loss / fat loss
	• lower blood pressure
	• lower cholesterol count

The TV Watcher's Workout is a beginner's exercise program designed for the millions of Americans who do not currently exercise but should begin exercising for health reasons. You can do this workout either watching television during the commercial breaks or you can incorporate all the exercises into one continuous session and receive a full-body workout in as little as 12 minutes. You will probably find the beginner's workouts easier than previous workouts you have tried. The exercises are simple but effective. You do not have to be in pain for a workout to be beneficial. You'll have to ignore that old adage, "No pain, no gain!"

The biggest difference between this workout and others you have seen or tried is that this workout requires no equipment (except maybe a few things you'll find in the kitchen). You won't need any expensive machines, no weights; just this easy-to-use book where each exercise is clearly demonstrated. You don't even need a television.

So, if you are one of the 40 percent of Americans who does not exercise and have not exercised in 10, 20, or even 30 years—this workout is for you!

Budgeting Time for Fitness

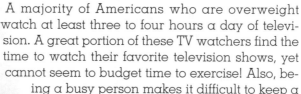

A majority of Americans who are overweight watch at least three to four hours a day of television. A great portion of these TV watchers find the time to watch their favorite television shows, yet cannot seem to budget time to exercise! Also, being a busy person makes it difficult to keep a workout schedule, but we all know that it is of utmost importance to get fit for health reasons.

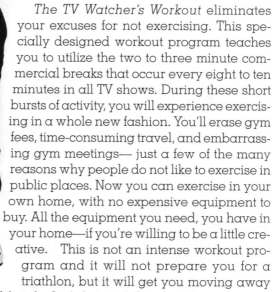

The TV Watcher's Workout eliminates your excuses for not exercising. This specially designed workout program teaches you to utilize the two to three minute commercial breaks that occur every eight to ten minutes in all TV shows. During these short bursts of activity, you will experience exercising in a whole new fashion. You'll erase gym fees, time-consuming travel, and embarrassing gym meetings— just a few of the many reasons why people do not like to exercise in public places. Now you can exercise in your own home, with no expensive equipment to buy. All the equipment you need, you have in your home—if you're willing to be a little creative. This is not an intense workout program and it will not prepare you for a triathlon, but it will get you moving away from your sedentary lifestyle. Let's face it, folks —you have to exercise every day to be healthy. Exercising can be as easy as walking, biking, skating or calisthenics. Just getting out of your Lazy-Boy Recliner for a total of 10-20 minutes a day can start the most sedentary person off on a lifelong pursuit of fitness and health. When trying to budget time for working out, just remember:

> Don't change your lifestyle to work out,
> change your workout to fit your lifestyle!

Top 10 Excuses for Not Exercising

1. Too busy (work, home, kids)
2. Takes too much time
3. Don't know how
4. Don't like gyms!
5. Too expensive
6. Don't look good in sweat clothes
7. Never have exercised before—why start now?
8. Can't stay motivated to continue a program
9. When weather stays cold, I stay indoors most of the time
10. I hate being sore!

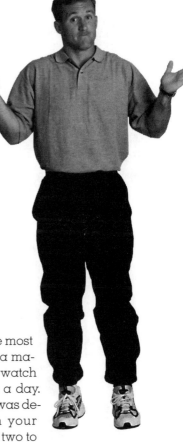

Is this Workout for Me?

This exercise program is designed for the most sedentary of us. We've just learned that a majority of the people who do not exercise watch at least three to four hours of television a day. So, you couch-commandos, if a workout was designed that would not interfere with your lifestyle, would you get up and move for two to three minutes at a time? I'm not talking about moving to the refrigerator either! You'll have to actually exercise different groups of muscles throughout your favorite TV shows. This is it! You can work out your entire body during a 30-minute television show during the four commercial breaks, each lasting only two to three minutes. Whether young or old, male or female, everyone can benefit from a workout that is designed to isolate each muscle group for maximum physical benefit.

Remember, this workout is not intended to train you for a triathlon, nor is it a quick way to a perfect body. It is designed to help you reach a healthy fitness level without impacting your comfortable or busy schedule.

TV is America's favorite pastime. Now you can take advantage of those commercials and get some exercise. After all, you have a lot of time.

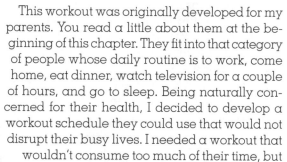

 that there are approximately 10 to 12 minutes of commercials in a 30-minute sitcom and 20 minutes of commercials in an hour-long show?

 that all you need to maintain a healthy lifestyle is 10 to 20 minutes of exercise a day?

 that you can effectively exercise every major muscle group in only 10 to 20 minutes?

 that effective workouts do not have to be continuous workouts? You can break up your workout throughout the day!

This workout was originally developed for my parents. You read a little about them at the beginning of this chapter. They fit into that category of people whose daily routine is to work, come home, eat dinner, watch television for a couple of hours, and go to sleep. Being naturally concerned for their health, I decided to develop a workout schedule they could use that would not disrupt their busy lives. I needed a workout that wouldn't consume too much of their time, but would inspire them to exercise and work toward a healthier lifestyle. They have never felt better. Their excuse for not exercising was that they couldn't find the time. Well, their problem has been remedied!

These exercises are derived from the exercises I learned during Navy SEAL training. I hope you will find the workouts easy to follow and sufficiently challenging.

So there you have it. A workout you can do in the privacy of your own home, at any time, during your favorite TV shows. You do not need to buy a single piece of equipment. All the gear you need is already in your home. You can use this workout all year long, during soap operas, game shows, comedies, news broadcasts, and sports shows. *The TV Watcher's Workout* is ideal for any lifestyle.

"But I Haven't Exercised In Years!"

Even if you have not exercised for several years, it won't take long for you to see the results of a steady exercise program. Steady exercise will help you achieve and maintain a basic level of fitness. Here are some goals to strive for:

1) **Increased flexibility.** By warming and stretching your muscles several times a week, you will be able to bend and touch body parts that you may not have touched in years!

2) **Improved muscle tone.** By performing resistance exercises, you'll become stronger and leaner.

3) **Decreased body fat percentage.** When beginning an exercise program that incorporates resistance training, you will lose body fat and build muscle. (The best way to measure your progress is by measuring inches instead of weight loss.) Attention Ladies: Do not fear, you will not build bulging muscles by doing these lightweight, high-repetition workouts.

4) **Weight loss.** If you have a lot of weight to lose, beginning any exercise program will aid in weight reduction. This workout will help you lose weight, but more importantly, you'll increase your lean muscle mass. The more muscle you build, the more calories you will burn when you exercise. As you replace fat with lean muscle, you'll see your energy level go through the roof and your waist line drop by inches.

5) **Walking for 45 minutes.** This workout program will help you walk for 45 to 60 minutes without stopping. Eventually, you may even be able to run for the same amount of time! You will be amazed by the progress you can make once you have a solid foundation.

6) **Performing pushups.** The common denominator between men and women who can perform pushups or any other upper body exercise is simple —THEY PRACTICE! If you cannot do these exercises when you begin this program, you will soon if you practice doing negatives or the special exercises like knee and chair pushups.

Testing Yourself

A great way to test your physical strength is to periodically see how many pushups and crunches you can do in one minute. A fitness test should also include a walk or run timed event as well. Try walking a mile as fast as you can without stopping. On the next page is a scale you can use to check your level of fitness.

	Superb	Excellent	Fantastic	Good	Keep Working
Pushups	40+	25–40	11–25	5–10	under 5
Crunches	50+	40–50	30–39	15–29	under 15
1 mile walk (min.)	10	11	12	13	14
1 mile run * (min.)	8	9	10	11	12

*Eventually, you will be able to run. However, I do not recommend running too early in your exercise program. Take it easy and build up to running. You should walk for a few months prior to beginning a running program. If you are extremely overweight, wait until you have lost a majority of your body fat. You can cause serious joint injuries by running when you are too heavy. Walking fast is a better fat-burning exercise anyway.

How It Works

Here is a typical scenario that will best describe how to use this workout. You'll be working out one of the four muscles groups on each commercial break. During this break, you'll cover every aspect of that muscle group, including stretching. For example, if it's the upper body series, you'll do chest and shoulder stretches, plus pushups, dips, curls, and arm kickbacks. You'll work out three days a week this way (say Monday, Wednesday, and Friday). On Tuesday and Thursday you're free to not work out, or better yet, to engage in some cardiovascular exercise such as walking or running. We'll talk more about those options later.

Back to Monday, and the workout. After your favorite TV show begins, there will be a two to three minute commercial break after the introduction. As the commercials begin, perform the stretches listed in the workout charts for commercial break number one. (Don't worry too much about the specific stretches and exercises now; we'll cover each commercial segment in depth in Chapter 4.)

After you've finished stretching (about 30 to 40 seconds), you will spend the next one and a half minutes performing exercises for that segment. When you're finished and your show's back on, sit back down, drink a glass of water, and wait for the next commercial series.

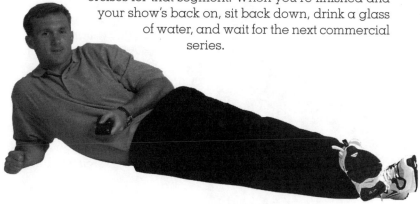

As You Increase Your Fitness Level

When you use the *TV Watcher's Workout*, you'll receive a choice of three workout programs: the pre-beginner's workout, the beginner's workout and the post-beginner's workout. Your goal should be to start with the level that matches your fitness ability, and work your way up to the post-beginner's workout. Eventually, I hope you won't need this workout at all, but will be able to move to longer, more intense workouts—away from the TV.

The **Pre-Beginner's Workout** is designed for those of you who have not exercised in years. During any 30-minute television show, there are four commercial series that last anywhere from two to three minutes. Simply do the exercises as they are outlined in the workout charts in Chapter Four. You will receive 10 to 12 minutes worth of exercise in this 30-minute time period. In each commercial break, you will focus on a different muscle group. For example, the first break will exercise your upper body muscles (arms, shoulders, and chest), while the second break will exercise the lower body muscles (legs, hips, and buttocks). The third commercial series focuses on the abdominal region (stomach and obliques). The fourth commercial series is gender specific; men will repeat the abdominal exercises, while women will do a series of hips, buttocks, and inner/outer thigh exercises.

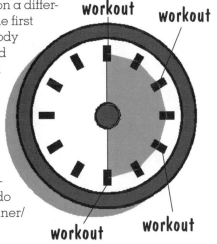

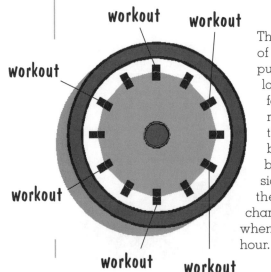

The **Beginner's Workout** is for those of you who need (or want) to be pushed a little longer. This workout lasts an hour and you will exercise for 20 minutes within this time period. The only difference between this workout and the pre-beginner's workout is that the beginner's workout lasts longer. Basically, you will perform two sets of the pre-beginner's workout. The chart to the left may help you visualize when you will be exercising during the hour.

The **Post-Beginner's Workout** is a continuous 12-minute workout. This one is for those days when you do not have the time to sit down and watch some TV, or when you've stop feeling challenged by the beginner's or pre-beginner's workouts. The great thing about this workout is that it can be accomplished anywhere—your house, office, and or hotel room. You don't need any equipment —just 12 minutes!

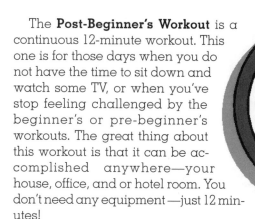

The chart below is an overview of the next twelve weeks:

TWELVE WEEK TV WATCHER'S WORKOUT			
	Workout Days	Off Days	All Days
Level 1 Wks 1–4	Pre-Beginner's Workout	Walk 10 min.	Stretch Before and After
Level 2 Wks 5–8	Beginner's Workout	Walk 20 min.	Stretch Before and After
Level 3 Wks 9–12	Post-Beginner's Workout	Walk or jog 20 min.	Stretch Before and After

My goal is to get America moving and away from the television. Exercising during the commercials is only the first step. It is my hope that eventually the workouts I've outlined here will be too easy, and your desire to exercise more strenuously will grow. I hope you'll someday put yourself in the former TV watcher's category.

So what are you waiting for? Let's begin!

CHAPTER TWO

Stretching

The most important thing to remember about exercising is that stretching is absolutely vital before you begin. The best way to stretch is to start at your head and end at your feet. Stretch each muscle for about 15 to 20 seconds before and after your workout. I've allotted you time during each commercial to stretch any muscles you have not exercised.

Stretching is important for a number of reasons:

 It relieves tension, which leads to head, back and neck aches.

 It prevents injuries by increasing the range of motion in your joints.

 It prepares the body for exercising by warming muscles and increasing the blood flow throughout the body.

Before you start any workout program, no matter how easy it appears, you should stretch daily for a full week to build flexibility. This is especially true if you have not exercised in a long time. Being flexible means you can move your body freely and without pain through a full range of motion. The chart on the next page is a guide for your week of pre-training. The chart lets you know how long each stretch should last and is a good way to keep track of your progress. It will only take you about ten minutes to completely stretch your entire body.

STRETCHING

2

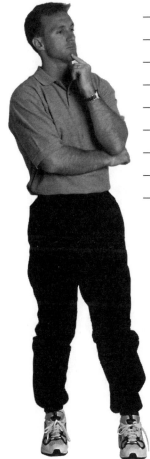

DAILY PRE-TRAINING STRETCHING WEEK	
STRETCHES	TIME
Neck	30 sec.
Shoulders	30 sec.
Chest	1 min.
Arms	1 min.
Stomach	1 min.
Legs	2 min.
Buttocks	1 min.
Full Body	30 sec.

If you have not exercised in several years, or ever, you should perform every stretch in this book for the allotted time on this chart for a full week—*before attempting any of the exercises!*

You will be less injury prone when you start to exercise and the soreness that accompanies newly exercised muscles will be decreased significantly. In less than ten minutes, you can stretch your entire body and feel better than ever.

A good stretch is one that is slow and easy with no bouncing motion. You should hold each stretch for about 15 to 20 seconds and repeat the stretch two to three times. You should never push a stretch to the point of pain. If you feel pain, relax! This is your body's way of indicating that something is wrong. It is recommended that you stretch every night before you go to sleep. For better results, you should stretch in the morning and evening.

So! You've just settled in after a long day at work. Your body is aching and you're ready for a couple of quality hours in front of the TV. Exercising hasn't even crossed your mind . . . If only you knew how easy it is to exercise—in front of the TV! Go ahead, try it—just reach up and stretch. Felt good, didn't it? Exercising will give you more energy, relieve tension, and doesn't have to interfere with your lifestyle. Convinced? Good. We'll start by stretching the neck.

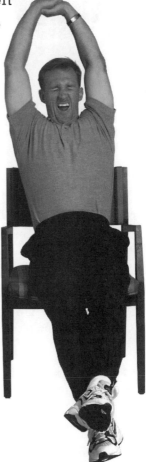

STRETCHING

2

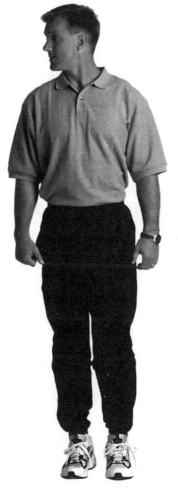

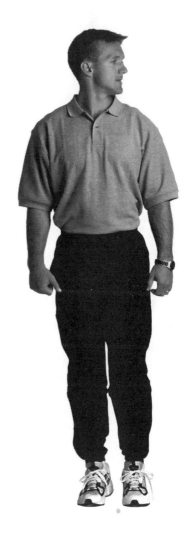

 ## Neck Stretches

Look to the left, right, up, and down, by turning your head slowly in these directions as shown. Your neck should move as if you were nodding "yes" and "no." Hold each motion for 15 seconds. Be careful! You do not want to raise, lower, or rotate your neck too much. You can cause severe neck injury this way, so be sure to always use slow and relaxing motions.

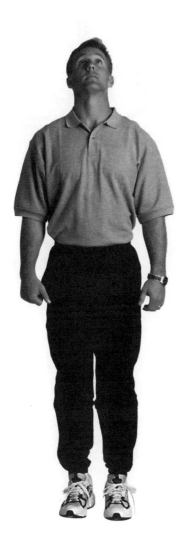

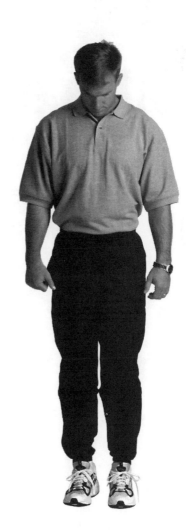

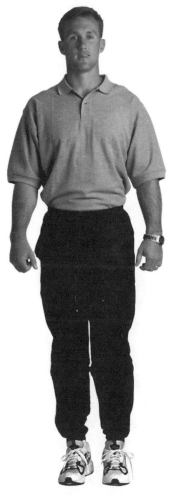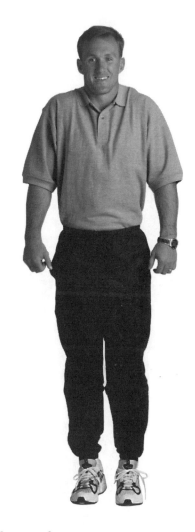

 ## Superbowl Shoulder Stretch

Rotate your shoulders slowly up and down, keeping your arms re-
laxed at your sides. This stretch will help relieve the pressure on the
base of your neck, keeping this area from tightening and causing
pain and headaches.

You will begin your stretching routine with neck and shoulder
stretches every day, but you can also use these stretches throughout
the day as tension builds. You can actually relieve or prevent headaches by simply keeping your neck and shoulders loose.

Arm Circles

From a standing or sitting position, rotate your arms slowly in big circles. This will loosen your shoulders and prepare them for exercises such as pushups, dips, and arm kickbacks. Arm circles are also good stress relievers, because they help relax the shoulder muscles that are connected to the base of your neck.

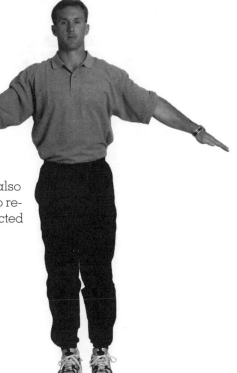

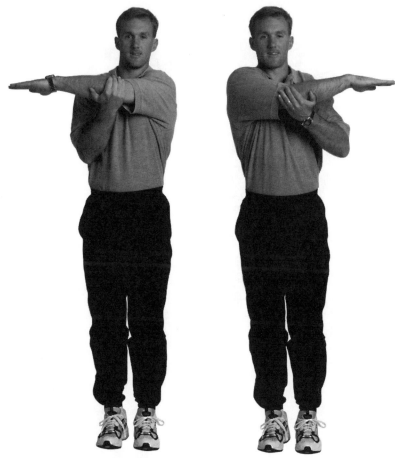

 ## Arm and Shoulder Stretch

Pull your right arm across your chest with your left hand placed on your right elbow as shown. Hold for 10 seconds, and then repeat with the other arm.

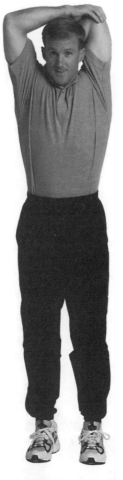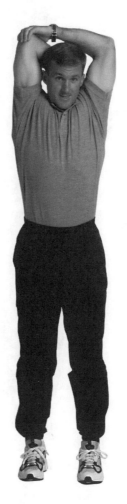

 ## Arms Like Arnold Stretch

Put both arms over and behind your head as shown. Grab your right elbow with your left hand and pull your elbow toward your opposite shoulder. Lean with the pull. Repeat with the other arm. You should hold this stretch for 15 seconds.

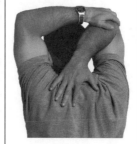

This stretch will help to stretch the triceps muscle, located in the back of the upper arm. You will firm this area by performing various types of pushups, dips, and isolation exercises.

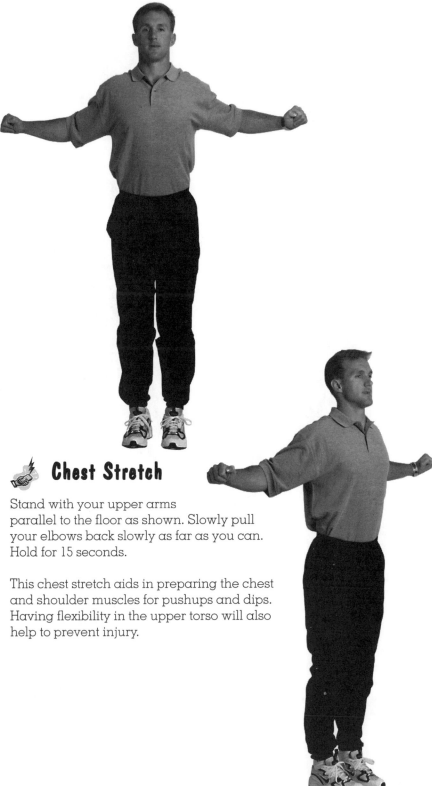

Chest Stretch

Stand with your upper arms parallel to the floor as shown. Slowly pull your elbows back slowly as far as you can. Hold for 15 seconds.

This chest stretch aids in preparing the chest and shoulder muscles for pushups and dips. Having flexibility in the upper torso will also help to prevent injury.

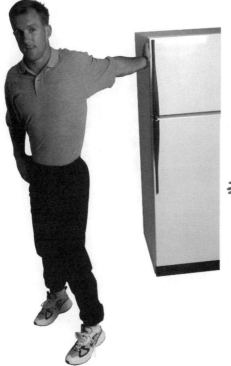

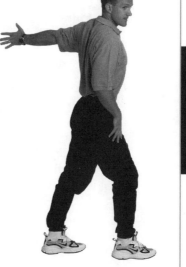

 ## Refrigerator Chest Stretch

The commercial's on and like many of us, you head straight for the kitchen. It's not that we're hungry, but there are so many good treats in there . . . You can avoid unnecessary snacking by performing this stretch instead.

Face away from the wall with one arm extended at shoulder level. Turn away slowly from the wall with your arm pushing against the wall as shown. Repeat the stretch with your other arm. You should stretch both arms for 10 seconds.

This is another effective method of stretching your chest and shoulder muscles. During your workout (or even if you're just a little tired or sore), choose which stretch works best for you and utilize it when needed.

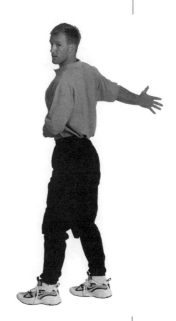

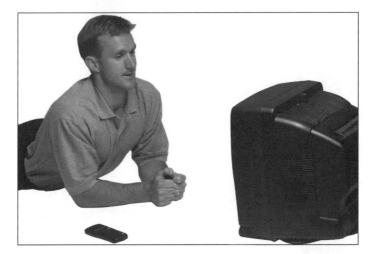

 ## Stomach Stretch

Lay on your stomach. Push yourself up on your elbows and leave your abdomen and legs flat on the ground. Slowly and carefully raise your head and shoulders. Be careful not to arch your back too much. Hold for 15 seconds and then repeat.

Before you perform any crunches, you need to thoroughly stretch your stomach muscles. This will help you achieve a full range of motion for any ab exercises.

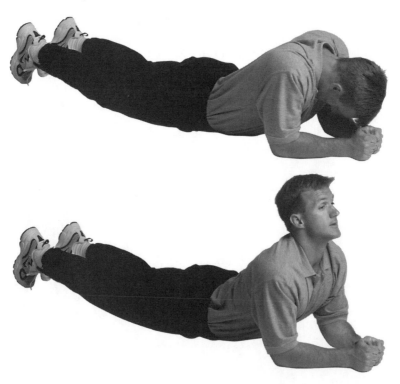

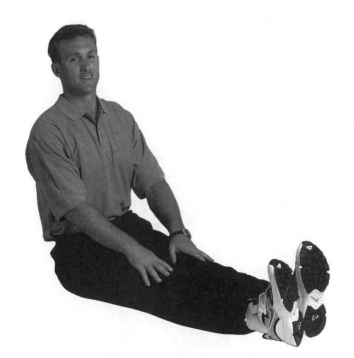

 ## Toe Touch

Sit on the floor with your legs in front of you. Lean toward your toes and grab your ankles. Hold for 15 seconds. Do not lock your knees!

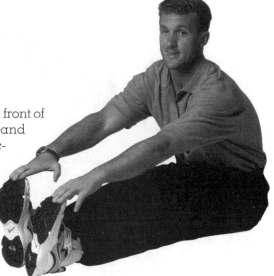

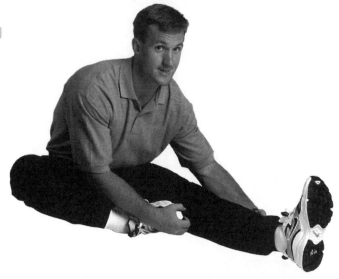

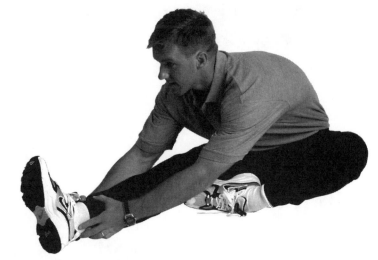

 ## Hurdler Stride

Sit on the floor with your legs straight in front of you. Bend your right knee and place the bottom of your foot on the inside of your opposite thigh. With your back straight, lean forward in order to stretch the back of your legs (hamstrings) and your lower back. Hold the stretch for 15 seconds.

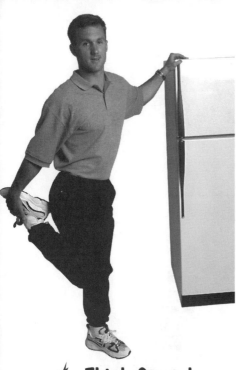

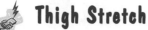 Thigh Stretch

Lay on your right side. Grab your left foot with your left hand and slowly pull your foot toward your buttocks. Hold the stretch for 15 seconds, and then switch sides. You can also perform this stretch standing, as shown.

It is important to keep your knees as close together as possible during this stretch. When performing leg exercises, you will need flexibility in your upper thigh area to reach a full range of motion and receive maximum benefits.

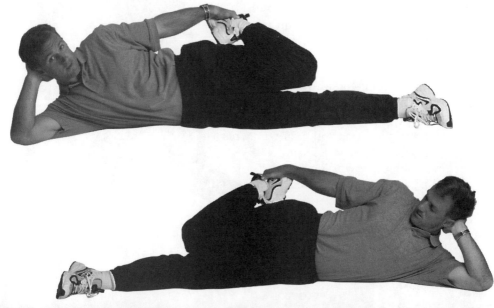

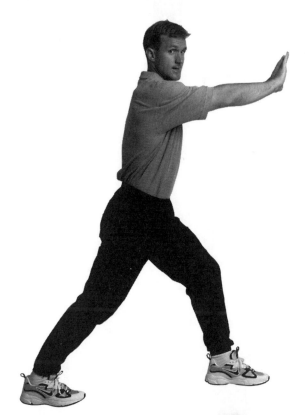

 ## Half-time Calf Stretch

Stand with one foot approximately two to three feet in front of your other foot in the stride position as shown. Bend your front leg forward, keeping your rear leg straight. Lean forward until you feel your rear calf muscle stretch. Make sure your toes are pointing in the direction you are facing. Hold for 15 seconds and repeat with the other leg.

As a modification of this exercise, and to stretch your Achilles tendon, simply bend your rear knee while in the same position as shown. This modification will completely stretch the lower leg and aid in preventing tendonitis in that area.

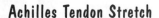

Achilles Tendon Stretch

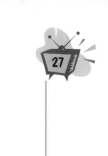
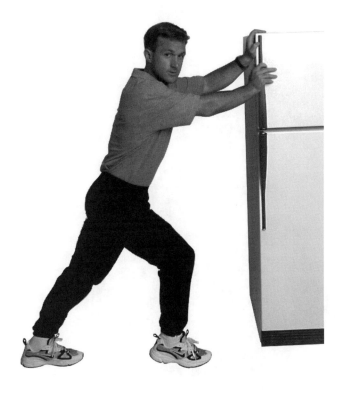

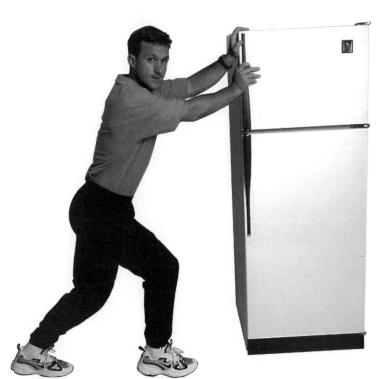

Achilles Tendon Stretch

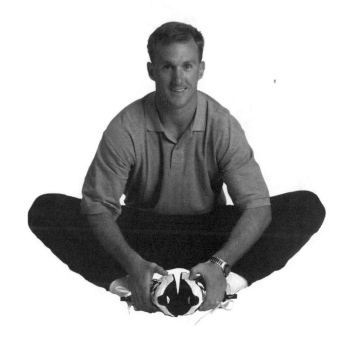

 Butterfly Stretch

Sit on your buttocks, with your legs bent and the soles of your feet together. Grab your ankles and place your elbows on your inner thighs. Slowly push down with your elbows.

This stretch helps to tone and loosen the inner thigh region. We'll use this stretch a lot in the Women's Workout prior to performing any inner thigh exercises.

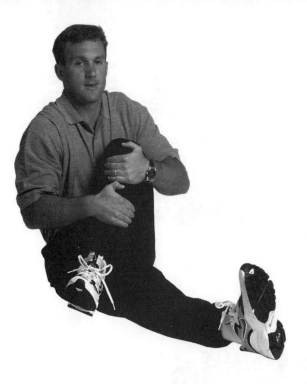

 # Hip / Buttocks Stretch

Sit on the ground with your legs crossed in front of you. Keeping your legs crossed, bring your right leg up so that your foot is placed flat on the ground next to your left knee. Pull your right leg all the way to your chest and hold for 15 seconds. Repeat with the other leg.

Before and after walking, running, or performing any lower body calisthenics exercises, make sure to properly stretch this tendon. This will prevent what is commonly known as "overuse injuries" in the hip and the knee. Keeping this area flexible is crucial to any fitness program.

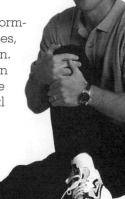

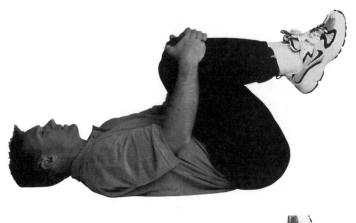

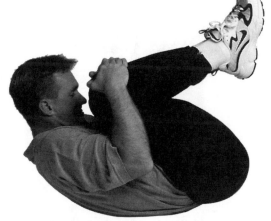

 ## Lower Back Stretch

Lay flat on your back. Pull your knees to your stomach region and hold with both arms as shown for 20 seconds. You should perform this stretch after completing the crunch exercises.

As you may know, the lower back is probably the most commonly injured area of the body. Many lower back strains are caused by inactivity, lack of flexibility, and overuse, such as lifting heavy objects improperly. Having an unusually large belly will also put an excessive strain on your back!

Full Body Stretch

Lay flat on the floor with your arms extended over your head and your lower back flat on the floor but not arched. Slowly stretch your entire body—try to make yourself an inch taller!

This is another great tension reliever after a tough day.

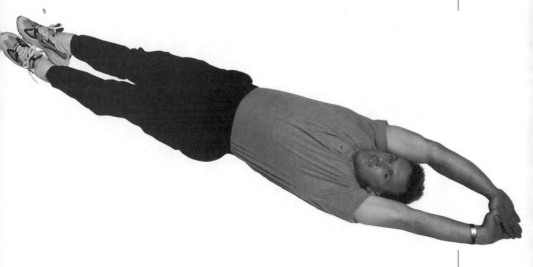

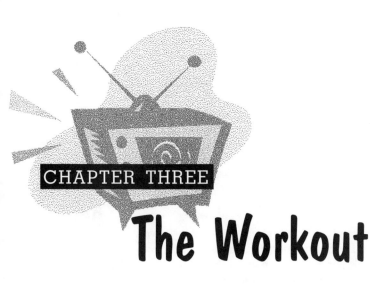

CHAPTER THREE

The Workout

This workout is designed to fit into the four series of commercial breaks, each lasting for an average of two to three minutes. I've included three levels of training with a four-week cycle for each level of progression. As the weeks add up, so do the repetitions of the exercises.

Television networks run approximately 20 minutes of commercials per hour. If you exercise for 20 minutes, you've gotten a great workout! The hardest part of any workout is finding the time and motivation to get started. Hopefully, you'll learn to take advantage of the commercial breaks during your favorite TV show. After all, you have already allotted the time to watch the show, and the commercials are hardly entertainment anyway. You can only benefit from utilizing this free time. It's really very easy.

You'll perform a series of exercises that isolate certain groups of muscles during each commercial break. Then rest, stretch, and watch your show. While you are exercising, you are naturally burning calories, but as you are resting you are burning calories too. This is due to an increased heart rate and blood flow to the recently exercised muscle group. This workout will help you build lean muscle mass and burn calories, fat, and inches in isolated areas of your body. Best of all, this is a full body workout.

You will find that two to three minutes of continuous exercise with the same muscle group is challenging. If you doubt this, try performing two to three minutes of pushups or situps. I think you'll change your mind!

There are three different workouts you can choose to do:

1. **Pre-Beginner's Workout (12 minutes):**
   Performed during any 30-minute
   television show.

2. **Beginner's Workout (20 minutes):** Performed during an hour long show or two
   30-minute shows. The only difference
   between this workout and the 12-Minute
   Workout is that in the 20-Minute
   Workout, you'll
   repeat each exercise twice.

3. **Post-Beginner's Workout (12 minutes
   continuously):** This one can be done without
   the TV! If you don't have the time to watch
   even one show, do each exercise continuously, without resting. It only takes 10
   to 12 minutes to get a full-body workout.

The workouts are organized to exercise the
four major muscle groups (conveniently the number
of commercial breaks in a 30-minute show). Here are
the four groups:

1. **Arms, Chest, and Shoulders**
   Exercises include: Chair dips, chair and knee
   pushups, arm kickbacks, and dumbbell curls

2. **Legs: Thighs, Hamstrings, and Calves**
   Exercises include: Squats, lunges, and heel
   raises

3. **Hips, Buttocks, and Inner Thighs**
   Exercises include: Pelvic lifts and leg lifts

4. **Abdominals and Obliques**
   Exercises include: Four-way crunches, oblique situps, and
   love handles

   PLEASE NOTE: In the early weeks of the workout, you may have extra
   time left before your show returns. In order to get the most out of your
   allotted time for exercising, you can repeat the exercises until the commercials are finished, walk in place, or do jumping jacks. Be creative!

After you've completed Level I, if you feel the need to challenge
yourself further, advance to Levels II and III. If you're not quite ready
for the next level, choose a week in Level I where you feel comfortable and repeat the cycle from there. Levels II and III are more challenging, but they are still easy enough to do during the two to three
minute commercial breaks.

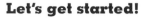

Let's get started!

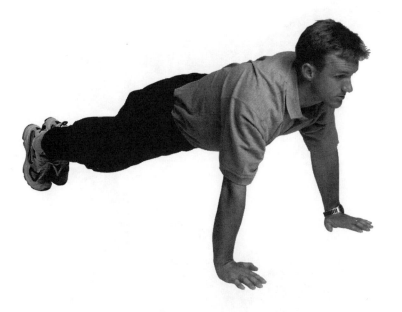

 ## Regis Regular Pushups

If you are able to do a regular pushup, that's great. Regular pushups are challenging and will work your chest muscles strenuously. Pushups are a great upper body exercise that will firm and strengthen your arms, shoulders, and chest.

Lay on the ground with your hands placed flat next to your chest. Push yourself up by straightening your arms and keeping your back straight.

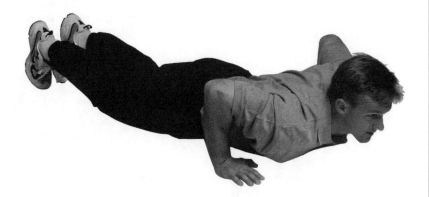

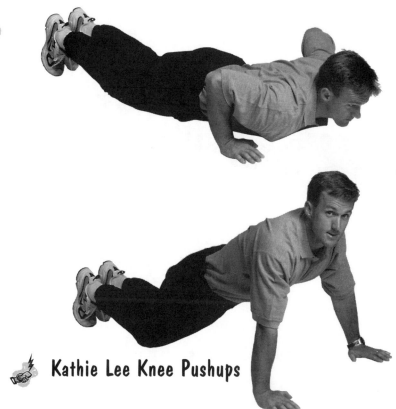

Kathie Lee Knee Pushups

Maybe you haven't done a pushup since gym class in high school, and you're a little out of practice. Try a knee pushup instead. Lay on your stomach with your hands on the floor next to your chest as shown. Keep your hands about shoulder width apart. With your knees on the ground, straighten your arms and push your body off the ground. Repeat.

If you cannot perform the required number of regular pushups, dropping to your knees will benefit the same muscles as regular pushups. Knee pushups are easier because they decrease the body weight placed on your arms.

A Word on Pushups

A common error when performing pushups is hand placement on the ground. Many beginners place their hands at or above shoulder height, which greatly decreases the range of motion of the arms and the ability to perform maximum repetitions. If you place your hands in the incorrect position shown here, you will place increased pressure on your shoulder joint, causing possible injury.

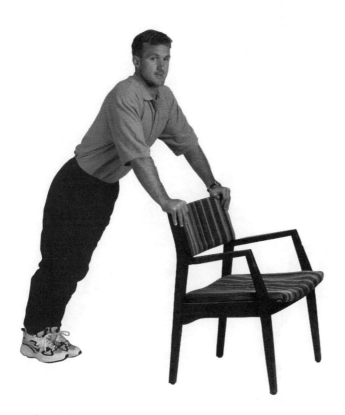

 ## Armchair Pushups

If you find that both knee and regular pushups are too difficult, don't give up! Try using a chair or table. Lean against the object with your feet together and push in the same fashion as a regular pushup. You'll still be working your chest muscles, and you'll be building your stamina to do regular pushups. Plus, there's the added benefit of being able to see the TV!

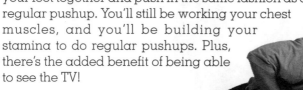

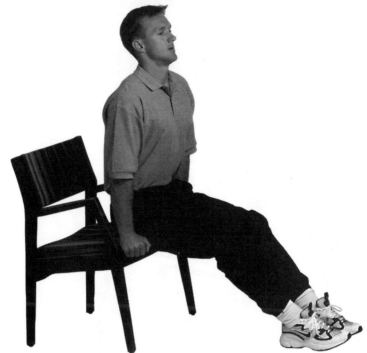

 ## Chips 'n Dips

Place your hands on the edge of your seat with your legs extended in front of you. Lower yourself until your elbows form a 90 degree angle as shown. Then straighten your arms and lift yourself back to your beginning level and repeat.

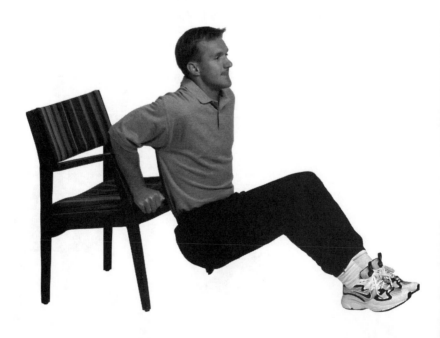

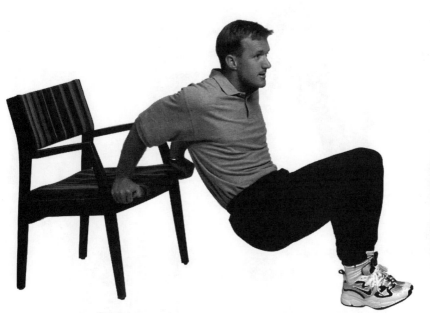

This incorrect position is sure to cause injury!

This exercise develops the triceps, chest, and shoulders. You must be careful not to hyper-extend your shoulders with this exercise, which you will do if you keep your arms straight or lower your body incorrectly as shown. This very common error can cause damage to your shoulder joints and chest muscles.

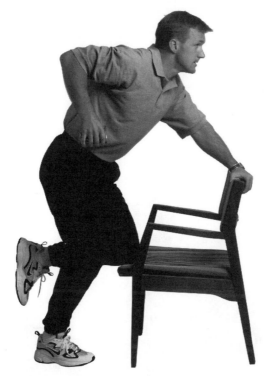

Arm Kickbacks

This exercise can be done with or without a dumbbell, but is best utilized with a little weight. Bend forward at the waist with one elbow tight at your side as shown. Fully straighten your arm behind you, flexing the back of your upper arm (your triceps muscle) at the top. Then form a 90 degree angle with your arm and repeat. Your arm shouldn't go any further than 90 degrees.

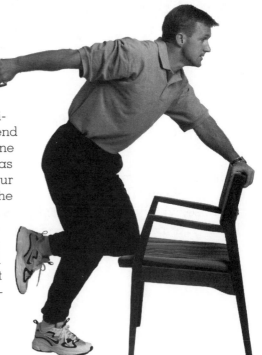

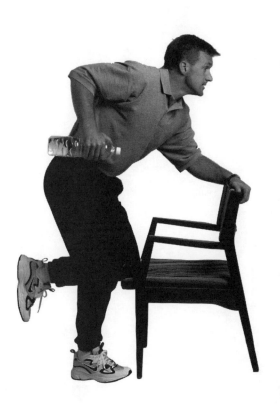

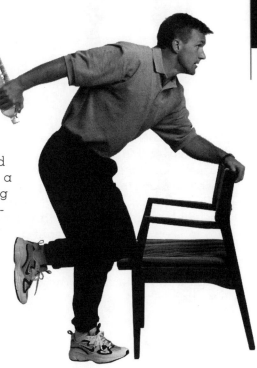

"Hey," you're thinking, "I thought I didn't need to buy any equipment!" You don't. Your fridge has all the equipment you need. Start out with a can of soup as your dumbbell. As you need to add more weight, try a bottle of water or something similar. Remember, be creative. It's your workout and you're in charge.

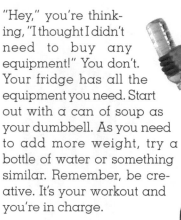

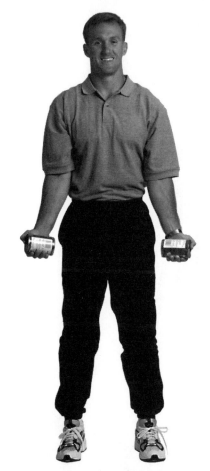

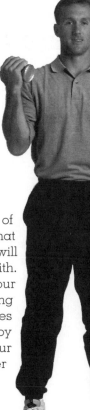

12 Oz. Curls

This exercise is best used with some type of weight as well. Make sure to pick a weight that you feel comfortable with, and one that you will be able to reach the required repetitions with. Stand up, keeping your elbows next to your sides and straightening your arms, making sure to keep your back straight and knees slightly bent. Lift your hands to your chest by bending your arms at the elbows, flexing your biceps when your hands are at shoulder level. Repeat.

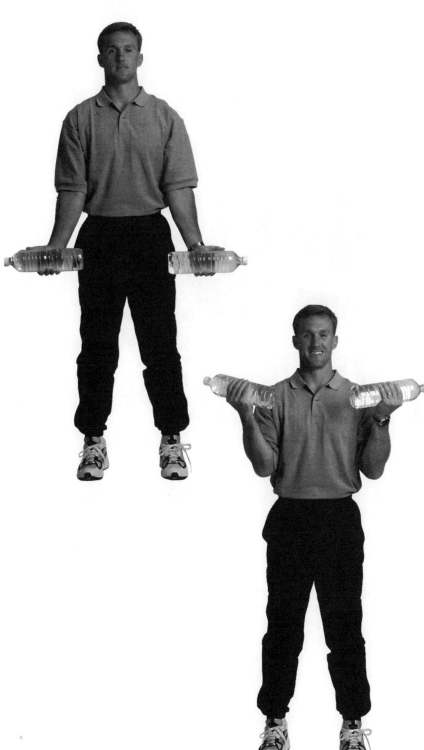

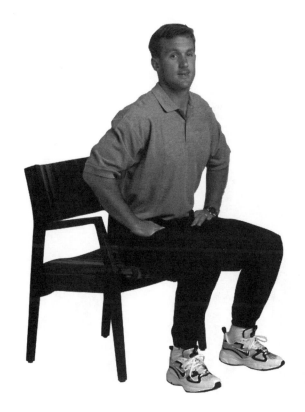

3

 ## Squats

Standing with your seat (or couch!) behind you, sit down and repeat the process of standing and sitting. Make sure that your back is straight (not arched), your head is up and your feet are about shoulder width apart. A good method to make sure your technique is correct is to look up at the ceiling while performing the exercise.

This exercise is excellent for toning your legs and buttocks. Make sure you perform this exercise flat-footed, trying not to go onto your toes when squatting, which places too much pressure on your knees and ankles. For the same reason, be careful not to bend your knees greater than 90 degrees. In order to stay flat-footed, try to spread your legs a little wider than shoulder width apart.

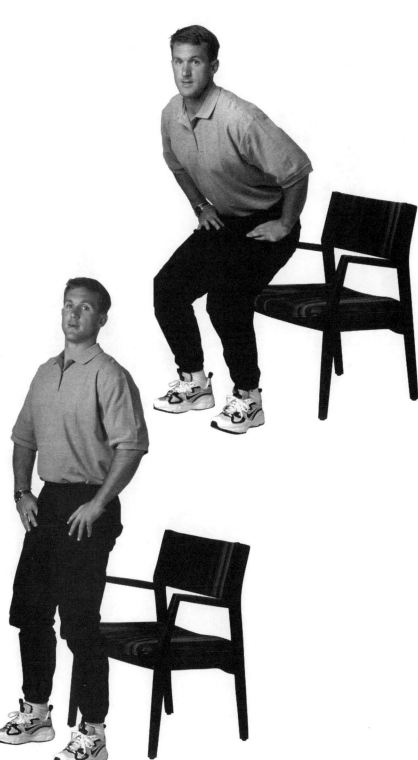

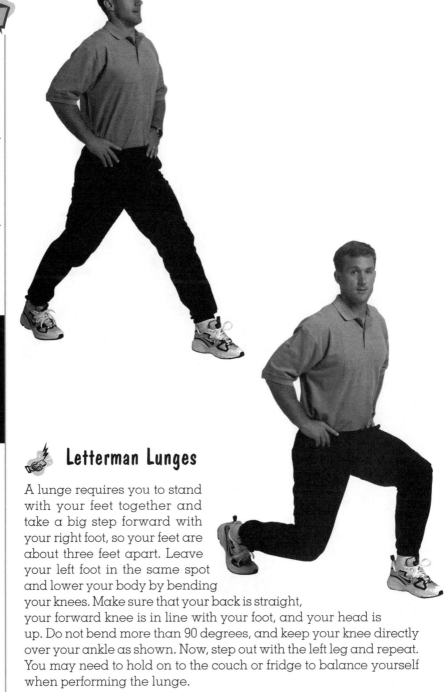

Letterman Lunges

A lunge requires you to stand with your feet together and take a big step forward with your right foot, so your feet are about three feet apart. Leave your left foot in the same spot and lower your body by bending your knees. Make sure that your back is straight, your forward knee is in line with your foot, and your head is up. Do not bend more than 90 degrees, and keep your knee directly over your ankle as shown. Now, step out with the left leg and repeat. You may need to hold on to the couch or fridge to balance yourself when performing the lunge.

If you have serious knee problems, the lunge may be too strenuous for you. If so, repeat the squat exercise instead of the lunge.

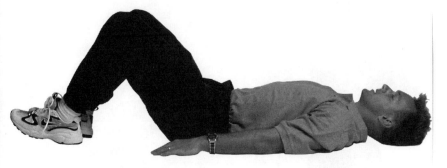

 ## Primetime Pelvic Lifts

Lay on your back with your knees bent and your feet and hands on the floor. Flex your buttocks as you lift your torso off the floor. Lower slowly and repeat. Your shoulders should remain flat on the ground throughout the exercise.

This exercise will help tone one of the primary problem areas for women: the buttocks, hips, and inner thighs. Each upward movement will flex these areas. For maximum benefit, hold the "up" position for three to five seconds before lowering your hips back to the ground.

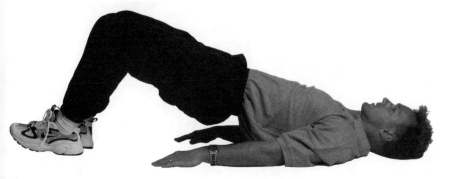

3

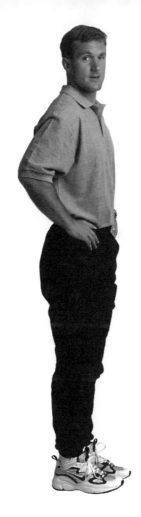

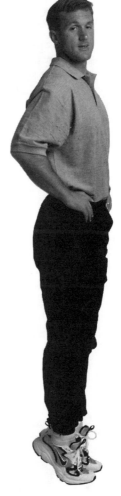

 ## Heel Raises

Stand up straight, place your feet together, and lean slightly against something to keep your balance. Lift yourself up onto your toes and back down slowly. (You can also perform this exercise one leg at a time as shown for a greater challenge.) Use a step or a stack of books to get full extension of the calf muscle. This exercise will tone your lower leg and strengthen your ankles.

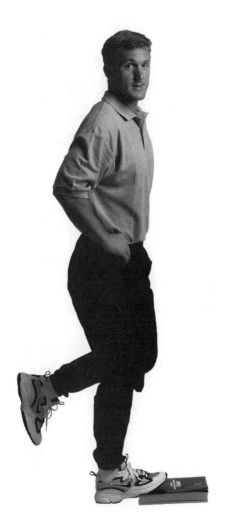

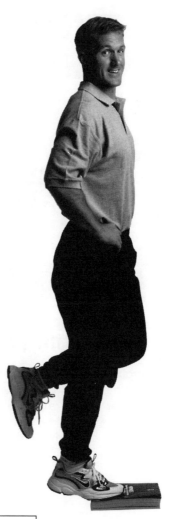

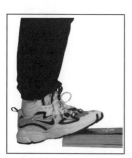

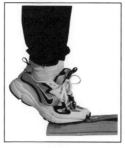

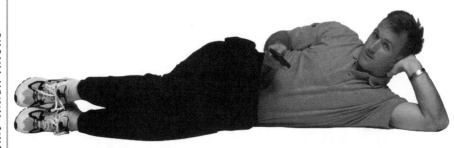

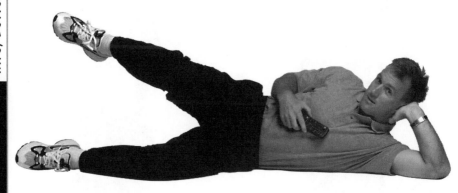

3

 ## Side Leg Lifts (Outer)

Lay on your right side with your knees slightly bent. Raise your top leg up as high as possible, usually about 18 to 24 inches off the ground. After you have completed the desired number of repetitions, roll over to your left side and repeat, raising your left leg. This exercise works the outer thigh muscles.

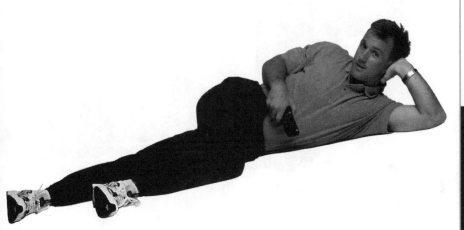

Side Leg Lifts (Inner)

Now, while in the same position on your side, place your top leg in front of your knee. Lift your bottom leg off the ground about 4 to 6 inches and repeat. This exercise will help tone and shape the inner thigh muscles.

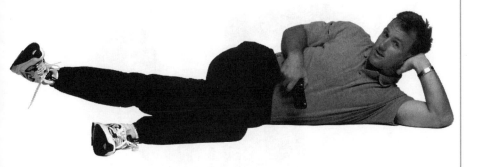

Brady Bunch Crunches

You will perform each crunch four ways: regular, left, right, and reverse. (In the workout charts, we'll refer to these as Four-Way Crunches.) This will allow you to work all the muscles in your abdomen equally for maximum benefit. We'll start with regular crunches.

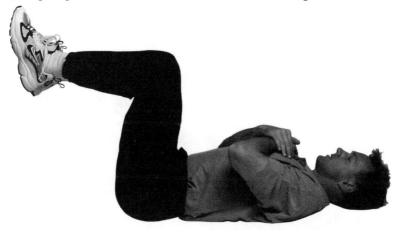

Regular

Lay on your back with your feet and knees in the air. (If you're really struggling, you can place your feet on the floor or use a chair to prop your feet up.) Cross your hands over your chest (not around your head) and bring your elbows to your knees.

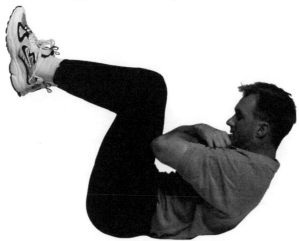

Brady Bunch Crunches (cont'd)

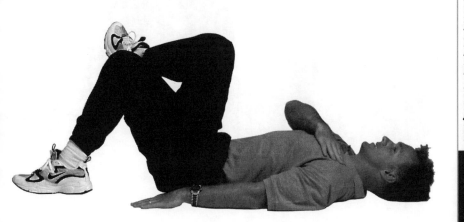

Right

In the same position, touch your right elbow to your left knee.

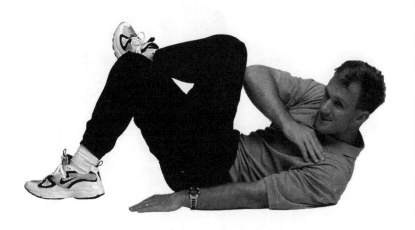

Brady Bunch Crunches (cont'd)

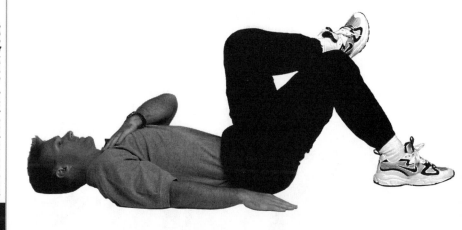

Left

Reversing the right crunch, touch your left elbow to your right knee.

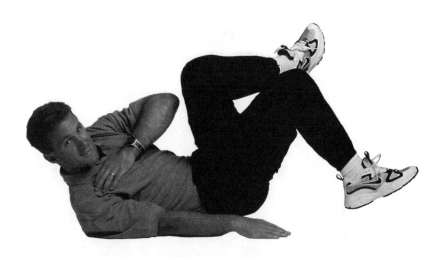

Brady Bunch Crunches (cont'd)

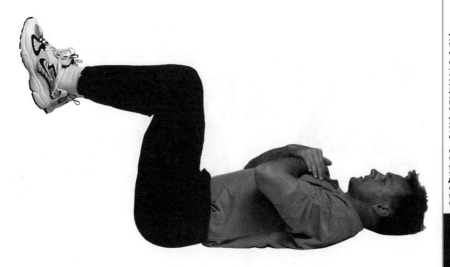

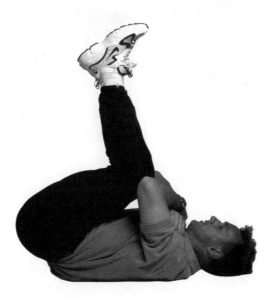

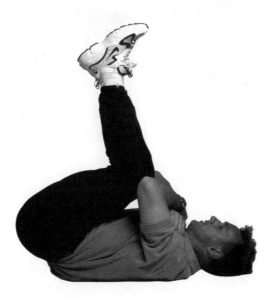

Reverse

Start in the same position. Instead of bringing your shoulders up as in the regular crunch, bring your knees to your elbows as shown. Leave your head on the ground. If you do the reverse crunch slowly and hold each crunch at the top, you'll get the best results.

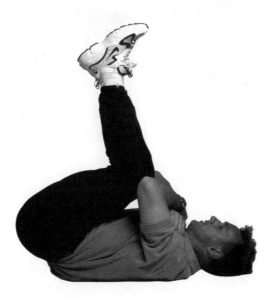

Brady Bunch Crunches (cont'd)

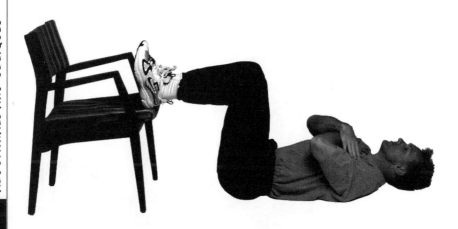

If it's too difficult to keep your feet in the air when performing crunches, try using a chair to prop your feet on.

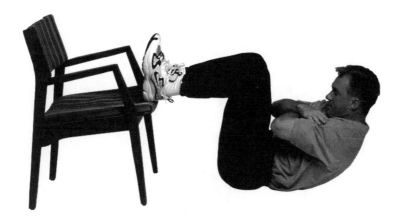

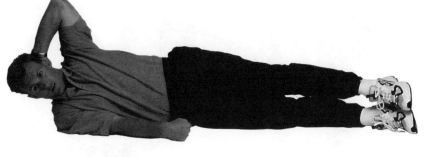

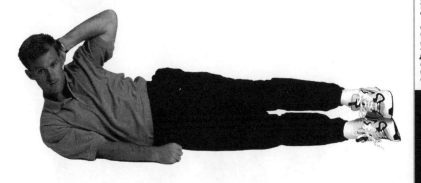

ABDOMINALS AND OBLIQUES

THE WORKOUT

3

 Oprah Obliques

Lay on the floor on your right hip and shoulder. Lift your feet about three inches off the ground, keeping your legs straight. (If this is too difficult, you can leave your legs on the floor.) Keeping your right arm tucked behind your neck as shown, slowly lift your right shoulder off the ground about two to three inches. You should feel this exercise working the sides of your torso just above your hips (your oblique muscles).

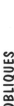

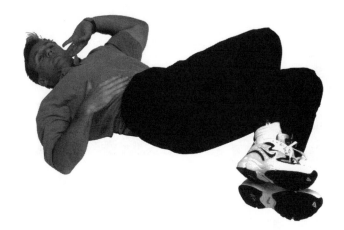

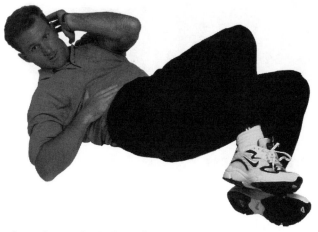

Loveboat Lovehandles

Lay on your back with your shoulders flat on the ground and your legs bent. Rotate your waist to the right, leaving your shoulders on the ground. You should be laying on your right hip. Slowly lift your upper body as shown as if you were doing a crunch. Repeat, then switch to the left side.

One of the problem areas for men are the lower left and right sides of the torso, better known as the "lovehandles." The best way to firm the muscles underneath the lovehandles is by performing a series of left and right side crunches or oblique situps. To get rid of the fat which make up the lovehandles, increase your heart rate by walking or biking in place. You have to move and eat sensibly in order to burn fat!

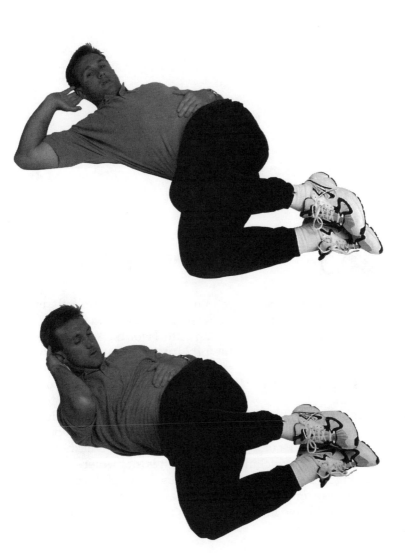

Men and women with big stomachs (or "potbellies") typically have lower back problems. The reason why is because the extra weight on your belly puts pressure on your lower back. That belly is the same as carrying 10, 20, or even 30 pounds around all day in your arms. Your lower back is weakened even more by lack of abdominal exercise. Developing your stomach muscles by doing crunches will help your posture and balance the opposing muscles of your lower back. Stretching and performing the back extensions in this workout will further develop your lower back muscles, decreasing your lower back pain.

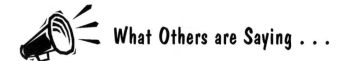 **What Others are Saying . . .**

Stew and I recently had our first child, Mary Elizabeth, in December of 1997. I gained over 60 pounds during the pregnancy. Within 5 months of giving birth, I was back to my pre-pregnancy weight using the program Stew developed for me. The same exercises, stretches and repetitions that are in the *The TV Watcher's Workout* helped me to look and feel fit again.

With a new child, I did not have a lot of time to exercise, so I used the workout for only 15 minutes at a time and could not believe the results. Walking in place, doing calisthenics exercises, and stretching—along with lots of water—really helped to burn fat and make my muscles more firm. If you do the program and stick to it for a few months, you will see the results!! Have fun—it is the easiest workout I have ever done in my life.

Denise Smith

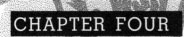
CHAPTER FOUR

Workout Schedules

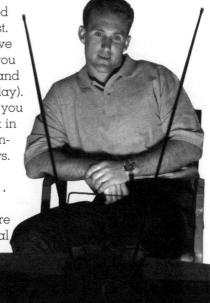

You will do one workout three times a week and then advance to a slightly more challenging one. There are three levels, and four weeks in each level, for a total of twelve weeks. On days in between the workouts, instead of doing nothing, you can walk in place and work your stomach muscles during the commercials.

The workout is designed to be utilized five days a week, with two days of rest. However, it is also perfectly fine to give yourself a day or two off, if you feel you need a break. You'll work out Days 1, 3, and 5 (say Monday, Wednesday, and Friday). Days 2 and 4 (Tuesday and Thursday) you can do a quick abdominal set or walk in place. Days 6 and 7 (Saturday and Sunday) are your resting and stretching days.

Let's walk through the first workout . . .

After your favorite TV show begins, there will be a two to three minute commercial break after the introduction. As the commercials begin, perform the stretches listed in the workout charts for commercial break number one, which will focus on your upper body. They are as follows:

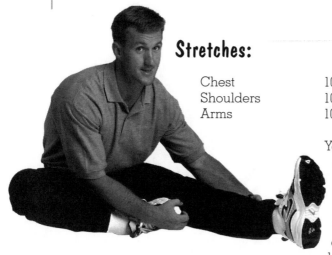

Stretches:

Chest	10 seconds
Shoulders	10 seconds
Arms	10 seconds each arm

You should pick whichever chest, shoulder, and arm stretch you feel most comfortable with, but try to vary them from workout to workout. You have only spent about a minute stretching. Now, in the next one and a half minutes, you will perform the following upper body exercises:

Exercises:

Pushups
Dips
Arm Kickbacks
Curls

The number of repetitions will depend on what week of the workout you are on. For example, in Level One, Week One you'll do 1–3 pushups, while in Level One, Week Four you'll do 4–6 pushups. These exercises will tone your shoulders, chest, and arms.

After you're finished, you can sit back down, drink a glass of water, and watch your show. Wait for the next commercial break, when we'll do abdominal stretches and exercises.

- **Stretch:**   Stomach Stretch   15 seconds
- **Exercises:**   Four-Way Crunches*
  Oblique Situps
  or Lovehandles

*A Four-Way crunch is one regular crunch, one reverse, one left and one right crunch. Remember, if you're doing 4 repetitions of the Four-Way crunch, that's four crunches each way!

These exercises will help you lose your belly and the dreaded lovehandles. Stand by for the next commercial segment, leg stretches and exercises:

- **Stretches:**
  Toe Touch 10 seconds
  Thigh Stretch 10 seconds each leg
  Calf Stretch 10 seconds each leg
- **Exercises:**
  Squats
  Lunges
  Heel Raises

The fourth commercial series will differ for men and women. We'll focus on trouble spots: hips and thighs for women and stomach and obliques for men. For women, the fourth commercial break is as follows:

- **Stretches:**
  Buttocks/ Hip Stretch 10 seconds each leg
  Butterfly Stretch 10 seconds
- **Exercises:**
  Pelvic Lifts
  Side Leg Lifts (inner)
  Side Leg Lifts (outer)

The men's workout for the fourth commercial series will concentrate on the stomach, including the sides of the torso (lovehandles):

- **Stretches:** Stomach Stretch
- **Exercises:** Four-Way Crunches
  Oblique Situps

Once you have finished the workout, you have two options:

1. Repeat the TV Watcher's Workout to receive the 20-Minute Workout
2. Relax and slowly stretch your muscles from head to toe.

On Tuesday and Thursday (or whenever your off days are), you should try to do some kind of cardiovascular exercise. Simply walk in place or ride a stationary bike while you watch TV. If continuous walking or biking is too difficult, you can start out by moving only during the commercials as you did with the calisthenics exercises. You can still benefit from two to three minute intervals of walking in a half hour or hour period. Eventually, you'll be able to walk uninterrupted for 20 or even 30 minutes.

Women's Workout starts on the next page;
Men's Workout begins on page 76.

WORKOUT SCHEDULES

4

MONDAY • WEDNESDAY • FRIDAY

 1st Commercial Break:

• Upper Body Stretches:	Neck	10 seconds
	Chest	10 seconds
	Shoulders	10 seconds
	Arms	10 seconds each arm
• Upper Body Exercises:	Pushups	1–3 reps
	Dips	1–3 reps
	Arm Kickbacks	5 reps each arm
	Arm Curls	5 reps each arm

 2nd Commercial Break:

• Ab Stretch:	Stomach Stretch	15 seconds
	Lower Back	15 seconds
• Ab Exercises:	Four-Way Crunches	5–8 reps
	Oblique Situps	5 reps each side
	or Lovehandles	5 reps each side

 3rd Commercial Break:

• Leg Stretches:	Toe Touch	10 seconds
	or Hurdler Stretch	10 seconds each leg
	Thigh Stretch	10 seconds each leg
	Calf Stretch	10 seconds each leg
• Leg Exercises:	Squats	5–8 reps
	Lunges	3–5 reps each leg
	Heel Raises	8 reps each leg

4th Commercial Break:

• Hip and Buttocks Stretches:	Hips/Buttocks Stretch	10 seconds each leg
	Butterfly Stretch	10 seconds
• Hip and Buttocks Exercises:	Pelvic Lifts	10 reps
	Side Leg Lifts (inner)	10 reps each leg
	Side Leg Lifts (outer)	10 reps each leg

After you've finished the workout, lie down and perform a full body stretch. It should feel great!

TUESDAY • THURSDAY

• Head-to-Toe Stretches: 10 minutes total

• Your choice cardiovascular exercise (walk in place during the commercials or for 10 to 20 minutes continuously)

MONDAY • WEDNESDAY • FRIDAY

1ST COMMERCIAL BREAK:

• Upper Body Stretches:	Neck	10 seconds
	Chest	10 seconds
	Shoulders	10 seconds
	Arms	10 seconds each arm
• Upper Body Exercises:	Pushups	2–4 reps
	Dips	2–4 reps
	Arm Kickbacks	6 reps each arm
	Arm Curls	6 reps each arm

2ND COMMERCIAL BREAK:

• Ab Stretch:	Stomach Stretch	15 seconds
	Lower Back	15 seconds
• Ab Exercises:	Four-Way Crunches	6–9 reps
	Oblique Situps	6 reps each side
	or Lovehandles	6 reps each side

3RD COMMERCIAL BREAK:

• Leg Stretches:	Toe Touch	10 seconds
	or Hurdler Stretch	10 seconds each leg
	Thigh Stretch	10 seconds each leg
	Calf Stretch	10 seconds each leg
• Leg Exercises:	Squats	6–9 reps
	Lunges	4–6 reps each leg
	Heel Raises	9 reps each leg

4TH COMMERCIAL BREAK:

• Hip and Buttocks Stretches:	Hips/Buttocks Stretch	10 seconds each leg
	Butterfly Stretch	10 seconds
• Hip and Buttocks Exercises:	Pelvic Lifts	12 reps
	Side Leg Lifts (inner)	11 reps each leg
	Side Leg Lifts (outer)	11 reps each leg

• **Don't forget your full body stretch!** •

TUESDAY • THURSDAY

• Head-to-Toe Stretches: 10 minutes total

• Your choice cardiovascular exercise (walk in place during the commercials or for 10 to 20 minutes continuously)

MONDAY • WEDNESDAY • FRIDAY

 ### 1ST COMMERCIAL BREAK:

• Upper Body Stretches:	Neck	10 seconds
	Chest	10 seconds
	Shoulders	10 seconds
	Arms	10 seconds each arm
• Upper Body Exercises:	Pushups	3–5 reps
	Dips	3–5 reps
	Arm Kickbacks	7 reps each arm
	Arm Curls	7 reps each arm

 ### 2ND COMMERCIAL BREAK:

• Ab Stretch:	Stomach Stretch	15 seconds
	Lower Back	15 seconds
• Ab Exercises:	Four-Way Crunches	7–10 reps
	Oblique Situps	7 reps each side
	or Lovehandles	7 reps each side

 ### 3RD COMMERCIAL BREAK:

• Leg Stretches:	Toe Touch	10 seconds
	or Hurdler Stretch	10 seconds each leg
	Thigh Stretch	10 seconds each leg
	Calf Stretch	10 seconds each leg
• Leg Exercises:	Squats	7–10 reps
	Lunges	5–7 reps each leg
	Heel Raises	10 reps each leg

 ### 4TH COMMERCIAL BREAK:

• Hip and Buttocks Stretches:	Hips/Buttocks Stretch	10 seconds each leg
	Butterfly Stretch	10 seconds
• Hip and Buttocks Exercises:	Pelvic Lifts	14 reps
	Side Leg Lifts (inner)	12 reps each leg
	Side Leg Lifts (outer)	12 reps each leg

• **Don't forget your full body stretch!** •

TUESDAY • THURSDAY

• Head-to-Toe Stretches: 10 minutes total

• Your choice cardiovascular exercise (walk in place during the commercials or for 10 to 20 minutes continuously)

MONDAY • WEDNESDAY • FRIDAY

1ST COMMERCIAL BREAK:

• Upper Body Stretches:	Neck	10 seconds
	Chest	10 seconds
	Shoulders	10 seconds
	Arms	10 seconds each arm
• Upper Body Exercises:	Pushups	4–6 reps
	Dips	4–6 reps
	Arm Kickbacks	8 reps each arm
	Arm Curls	8 reps each arm

2ND COMMERCIAL BREAK:

• Ab Stretch:	Stomach Stretch	15 seconds
	Lower Back	15 seconds
• Ab Exercises:	Four-Way Crunches	8–11 reps
	Oblique Situps	8 reps each side
	or Lovehandles	8 reps each side

3RD COMMERCIAL BREAK:

• Leg Stretches:	Toe Touch	10 seconds
	or Hurdler Stretch	10 seconds each leg
	Thigh Stretch	10 seconds each leg
	Calf Stretch	10 seconds each leg
• Leg Exercises:	Squats	8–11 reps
	Lunges	6–8 reps each leg
	Heel Raises	16 reps each leg

4TH COMMERCIAL BREAK:

• Hip and Buttocks Stretches:	Hips/Buttocks Stretch	10 seconds each leg
	Butterfly Stretch	10 seconds
• Hip and Buttocks Exercises:	Pelvic Lifts	15 reps
	Side Leg Lifts (inner)	13 reps each leg
	Side Leg Lifts (outer)	13 reps each leg

• **Don't forget your full body stretch!** •

TUESDAY • THURSDAY

• Head-to-Toe Stretches: 10 minutes total

• Your choice cardiovascular exercise (walk in place during the commercials or for 10 to 20 minutes continuously)

WOMEN'S WORKOUT

WORKOUT SCHEDULES

4

MONDAY • WEDNESDAY • FRIDAY

1st Commercial Break:

• Upper Body Stretches:	Neck	10 seconds
	Chest	10 seconds
	Shoulders	10 seconds
	Arms	10 seconds each arm
• Upper Body Exercises:	Pushups	9–12 reps
	Dips	9–12 reps
	Arm Kickbacks	9 reps each arm
	Arm Curls	9 reps each arm

2nd Commercial Break:

• Ab Stretch:	Stomach Stretch	15 seconds
	Lower Back	15 seconds
• Ab Exercises:	Four-Way Crunches	9–12 reps
	Oblique Situps	9 reps each side
	or Lovehandles	9 reps each side

3rd Commercial Break:

• Leg Stretches:	Toe Touch	10 seconds
	or Hurdler Stretch	10 seconds each leg
	Thigh Stretch	10 seconds each leg
	Calf Stretch	10 seconds each leg
• Leg Exercises:	Squats	9–12 reps
	Lunges	5–8 reps each leg
	Heel Raises	18 reps each leg

4th Commercial Break:

• Hip and Buttocks Stretches:	Hips/Buttocks Stretch	10 seconds each leg
	Butterfly Stretch	10 seconds
• Hip and Buttocks Exercises:	Pelvic Lifts	16 reps
	Side Leg Lifts (inner)	14 reps each leg
	Side Leg Lifts (outer)	14 reps each leg

• **Don't forget your full body stretch!** •

TUESDAY • THURSDAY

• Head-to-Toe Stretches: 10 minutes total

• Your choice cardiovascular exercise (walk in place during the commercials or for 10 to 20 minutes continuously)

MONDAY • WEDNESDAY • FRIDAY

 1ST COMMERCIAL BREAK:

• Upper Body Stretches:	Neck	10 seconds
	Chest	10 seconds
	Shoulders	10 seconds
	Arms	10 seconds each arm
• Upper Body Exercises:	Pushups	5–8 reps
	Dips	5–8 reps
	Arm Kickbacks	10 reps each arm
	Arm Curls	10 reps each arm

2ND COMMERCIAL BREAK:

• Ab Stretch:	Stomach Stretch	15 seconds
	Lower Back	15 seconds
• Ab Exercises:	Four-Way Crunches	10–13 reps
	Oblique Situps	10 reps each side
	or Lovehandles	10 reps each side

3RD COMMERCIAL BREAK:

• Leg Stretches:	Toe Touch	10 seconds
	or Hurdler Stretch	10 seconds each leg
	Thigh Stretch	10 seconds each leg
	Calf Stretch	10 seconds each leg
• Leg Exercises:	Squats	10–13 reps
	Lunges	6–9 reps each leg
	Heel Raises	18 reps each leg

4TH COMMERCIAL BREAK:

• Hip and Buttocks Stretches:	Hips/Buttocks Stretch	10 seconds each leg
	Butterfly Stretch	10 seconds
• Hip and Buttocks Exercises:	Pelvic Lifts	16 reps
	Side Leg Lifts (inner)	14 reps each leg
	Side Leg Lifts (outer)	14 reps each leg

• **Don't forget your full body stretch!** •

TUESDAY • THURSDAY

• Head-to-Toe Stretches: 10 minutes total

• Your choice cardiovascular exercise (walk in place during the commercials or for 10 to 20 minutes continuously)

WOMEN'S WORKOUT

WORKOUT SCHEDULES

4

MONDAY • WEDNESDAY • FRIDAY

1st Commercial Break:

• Upper Body Stretches:	Neck	10 seconds
	Chest	10 seconds
	Shoulders	10 seconds
	Arms	10 seconds each arm
• Upper Body Exercises:	Pushups	6–9 reps
	Dips	6–9 reps
	Arm Kickbacks	11 reps each arm
	Arm Curls	11 reps each arm

2nd Commercial Break:

• Ab Stretch:	Stomach Stretch	15 seconds
	Lower Back	15 seconds
• Ab Exercises:	Four-Way Crunches	10–13 reps
	Oblique Situps	12 reps each side
	or Lovehandles	12 reps each side

3rd Commercial Break:

• Leg Stretches:	Toe Touch	10 seconds
	or Hurdler Stretch	10 seconds each leg
	Thigh Stretch	10 seconds each leg
	Calf Stretch	10 seconds each leg
• Leg Exercises:	Squats	10–13 reps
	Lunges	6–9 reps each leg
	Heel Raises	19 reps each leg

4th Commercial Break:

• Hip and Buttocks Stretches:	Hips/Buttocks Stretch	10 seconds each leg
	Butterfly Stretch	10 seconds
• Hip and Buttocks Exercises:	Pelvic Lifts	18 reps
	Side Leg Lifts (inner)	16 reps each leg
	Side Leg Lifts (outer)	16 reps each leg

• **Don't forget your full body stretch!** •

TUESDAY • THURSDAY

• Head-to-Toe Stretches: 10 minutes total

• Your choice cardiovascular exercise (walk in place during the commercials or for 10 to 20 minutes continuously)

MONDAY • WEDNESDAY • FRIDAY

 ### 1ST COMMERCIAL BREAK:

- Upper Body Stretches:

Neck	10 seconds
Chest	10 seconds
Shoulders	10 seconds
Arms	10 seconds each arm

- Upper Body Exercises:

Pushups	6–9 reps
Dips	6–9 reps
Arm Kickbacks	12 reps each arm
Arm Curls	12 reps each arm

 ### 2ND COMMERCIAL BREAK:

- Ab Stretch:

Stomach Stretch	15 seconds
Lower Back	15 seconds

- Ab Exercises:

Four-Way Crunches	11–14 reps
Oblique Situps	13 reps each side
or Lovehandles	13 reps each side

 ### 3RD COMMERCIAL BREAK:

- Leg Stretches:

Toe Touch	10 seconds
or Hurdler Stretch	10 seconds each leg
Thigh Stretch	10 seconds each leg
Calf Stretch	10 seconds each leg

- Leg Exercises:

Squats	11–14 reps
Lunges	7–10 reps each leg
Heel Raises	20 reps each leg

 ### 4TH COMMERCIAL BREAK:

- Hip and Buttocks Stretches:

Hips/Buttocks Stretch	10 seconds each leg
Butterfly Stretch	10 seconds

- Hip and Buttocks Exercises:

Pelvic Lifts	18 reps
Side Leg Lifts (inner)	17 reps each leg
Side Leg Lifts (outer)	17 reps each leg

• **Don't forget your full body stretch!** •

TUESDAY • THURSDAY

- Head-to-Toe Stretches: 10 minutes total

- Your choice cardiovascular exercise (walk in place during the commercials or for 10 to 20 minutes continuously)

LEVEL ① ② ❸   WEEK ❶ ② ③ ④

MONDAY • WEDNESDAY • FRIDAY

 1st COMMERCIAL BREAK:

• Upper Body Stretches:	Neck	10 seconds
	Chest	10 seconds
	Shoulders	10 seconds
	Arms	10 seconds each arm
• Upper Body Exercises:	Pushups	7–10 reps
	Dips	7–10 reps
	Arm Kickbacks	13 reps each arm
	Arm Curls	13 reps each arm

 2nd COMMERCIAL BREAK:

• Ab Stretch:	Stomach Stretch	15 seconds
	Lower Back	15 seconds
• Ab Exercises:	Four-Way Crunches	12–15 reps
	Oblique Situps	14 reps each side
	or Lovehandles	14 reps each side

3rd COMMERCIAL BREAK:

• Leg Stretches:	Toe Touch	10 seconds
	or Hurdler Stretch	10 seconds each leg
	Thigh Stretch	10 seconds each leg
	Calf Stretch	10 seconds each leg
• Leg Exercises:	Squats	12–15 reps
	Lunges	8–10 reps each leg
	Heel Raises	21 reps each leg

4th COMMERCIAL BREAK:

• Hip and Buttocks Stretches:	Hips/Buttocks Stretch	10 seconds each leg
	Butterfly Stretch	10 seconds
• Hip and Buttocks Exercises:	Pelvic Lifts	19 reps
	Side Leg Lifts (inner)	18 reps each leg
	Side Leg Lifts (outer)	18 reps each leg

• **Don't forget your full body stretch!** •

TUESDAY • THURSDAY

• Head-to-Toe Stretches: 10 minutes total

• Your choice cardiovascular exercise (walk in place during the commercials or for 10 to 20 minutes continuously)

MONDAY • WEDNESDAY • FRIDAY

 ### 1ST COMMERCIAL BREAK:

- Upper Body Stretches:

Neck	10 seconds
Chest	10 seconds
Shoulders	10 seconds
Arms	10 seconds each arm

- Upper Body Exercises:

Pushups	8–11 reps
Dips	8–11 reps
Arm Kickbacks	14 reps each arm
Arm Curls	14 reps each arm

 ### 2ND COMMERCIAL BREAK:

- Ab Stretch:

Stomach Stretch	15 seconds
Lower Back	15 seconds

- Ab Exercises:

Four-Way Crunches	13–15 reps
Oblique Situps	15 reps each side
or Lovehandles	15 reps each side

 ### 3RD COMMERCIAL BREAK:

- Leg Stretches:

Toe Touch	10 seconds
or Hurdler Stretch	10 seconds each leg
Thigh Stretch	10 seconds each leg
Calf Stretch	10 seconds each leg

- Leg Exercises:

Squats	13–15 reps
Lunges	9–13 reps each leg
Heel Raises	22 reps each leg

 ### 4TH COMMERCIAL BREAK:

- Hip and Buttocks Stretches:

Hips/Buttocks Stretch	10 seconds each leg
Butterfly Stretch	10 seconds

- Hip and Buttocks Exercises:

Pelvic Lifts	20 reps
Side Leg Lifts (inner)	20 reps each leg
Side Leg Lifts (outer)	20 reps each leg

• **Don't forget your full body stretch!** •

TUESDAY • THURSDAY

- Head-to-Toe Stretches: 10 minutes total

- Your choice cardiovascular exercise (walk in place during the commercials or for 10 to 20 minutes continuously)

MONDAY • WEDNESDAY • FRIDAY

 1ST COMMERCIAL BREAK:

• Upper Body Stretches:	Neck	10 seconds
	Chest	10 seconds
	Shoulders	10 seconds
	Arms	10 seconds each arm
• Upper Body Exercises:	Pushups	9–12 reps
	Dips	9–12 reps
	Arm Kickbacks	15 reps each arm
	Arm Curls	15 reps each arm

 2ND COMMERCIAL BREAK:

• Ab Stretch:	Stomach Stretch	15 seconds
	Lower Back	15 seconds
• Ab Exercises:	Four-Way Crunches	18 reps
	Oblique Situps	16 reps each side
	or Lovehandles	16 reps each side

 3RD COMMERCIAL BREAK:

• Leg Stretches:	Toe Touch	10 seconds
	or Hurdler Stretch	10 seconds each leg
	Thigh Stretch	10 seconds each leg
	Calf Stretch	10 seconds each leg
• Leg Exercises:	Squats	14–17 reps
	Lunges	10–12 reps each leg
	Heel Raises	24 reps each leg

 4TH COMMERCIAL BREAK:

• Hip and Buttocks Stretches:	Hips/Buttocks Stretch	10 seconds each leg
	Butterfly Stretch	10 seconds
• Hip and Buttocks Exercises:	Pelvic Lifts	22 reps
	Side Leg Lifts (inner)	20 reps each leg
	Side Leg Lifts (outer)	20 reps each leg

• **Don't forget your full body stretch!** •

TUESDAY • THURSDAY

• Head-to-Toe Stretches: 10 minutes total

• Your choice cardiovascular exercise (walk in place during the commercials or for 10 to 20 minutes continuously)

MONDAY • WEDNESDAY • FRIDAY

 1ST COMMERCIAL BREAK:

• Upper Body Stretches:	Neck	10 seconds
	Chest	10 seconds
	Shoulders	10 seconds
	Arms	10 seconds each arm
• Upper Body Exercises:	Pushups	10–13 reps
	Dips	10–13 reps
	Arm Kickbacks	16 reps each arm
	Arm Curls	16 reps each arm

 2ND COMMERCIAL BREAK:

• Ab Stretch:	Stomach Stretch	15 seconds
	Lower Back	15 seconds
• Ab Exercises:	Four-Way Crunches	20 reps
	Oblique Situps	20 reps each side
	or Lovehandles	20 reps each side

 3RD COMMERCIAL BREAK:

• Leg Stretches:	Toe Touch	10 seconds
	or Hurdler Stretch	10 seconds each leg
	Thigh Stretch	10 seconds each leg
	Calf Stretch	10 seconds each leg
• Leg Exercises:	Squats	15–18 reps
	Lunges	10–13 reps each leg
	Heel Raises	25 reps each leg

 4TH COMMERCIAL BREAK:

• Hip and Buttocks Stretches:	Hips/Buttocks Stretch	10 seconds each leg
	Butterfly Stretch	10 seconds
• Hip and Buttocks Exercises:	Pelvic Lifts	25 reps
	Side Leg Lifts (inner)	20 reps each leg
	Side Leg Lifts (outer)	20 reps each leg

• **Don't forget your full body stretch!** •

TUESDAY • THURSDAY

• Head-to-Toe Stretches: 10 minutes total

• Your choice cardiovascular exercise (walk in place during the commercials or for 10 to 20 minutes continuously)

WOMEN'S WORKOUT

WORKOUT SCHEDULES

4

MONDAY • WEDNESDAY • FRIDAY

1ST COMMERCIAL BREAK:

• Upper Body Stretches:	Neck	10 seconds
	Chest	10 seconds
	Shoulders	10 seconds
	Arms	10 seconds each arm
• Upper Body Exercises:	Pushups	3–5 reps
	Dips	3–5 reps
	Arm Kickbacks	6 reps each arm
	Arm Curls	6 reps each arm

2ND COMMERCIAL BREAK:

• Ab Stretch:	Stomach Stretch	15 seconds
	Lower Back	15 seconds
• Ab Exercises:	Four-Way Crunches	5–8 reps
	Oblique Situps	5 reps each side
	or Lovehandles	5 reps each side

3RD COMMERCIAL BREAK:

• Leg Stretches:	Toe Touch	10 seconds
	or Hurdler Stretch	10 seconds each leg
	Thigh Stretch	10 seconds each leg
	Calf Stretch	10 seconds each leg
• Leg Exercises:	Squats	5–8 reps
	Lunges	3–5 reps each leg
	Heel Raises	8 reps each leg

4TH COMMERCIAL BREAK:

• Ab Stretch:	Stomach Stretch	15 seconds
• Stomach Exercises:	Four-Way Crunches	5–8 reps
	Oblique Situps	5–8 reps each side

• **Don't forget your full body stretch!** •

TUESDAY • THURSDAY

• Head-to-Toe Stretches: 10 minutes total

• Your choice cardiovascular exercise (walk in place during the commercials or for 10 to 20 minutes continuously)

MEN'S WORKOUT

WORKOUT SCHEDULES

4

MONDAY • WEDNESDAY • FRIDAY

 1ST COMMERCIAL BREAK:

- Upper Body Stretches:
	Neck	10 seconds
	Chest	10 seconds
	Shoulders	10 seconds
	Arms	10 seconds each arm

- Upper Body Exercises:
	Pushups	4–6 reps
	Dips	4–6 reps
	Arm Kickbacks	7 reps each arm
	Arm Curls	7 reps each arm

 2ND COMMERCIAL BREAK:

- Ab Stretch:
	Stomach Stretch	15 seconds
	Lower Back	15 seconds

- Ab Exercises:
	Four-Way Crunches	6–9 reps
	Oblique Situps	7 reps each side
	or Lovehandles	7 reps each side

 3RD COMMERCIAL BREAK:

- Leg Stretches:
	Toe Touch	10 seconds
	or Hurdler Stretch	10 seconds each leg
	Thigh Stretch	10 seconds each leg
	Calf Stretch	10 seconds each leg

- Leg Exercises:
	Squats	6–9 reps
	Lunges	4–6 reps each leg
	Heel Raises	9 reps each leg

 4TH COMMERCIAL BREAK:

- Ab Stretch:
	Stomach Stretch	15 seconds

- Stomach Exercises:
	Four-Way Crunches	6–9 reps
	Oblique Situps	6–9 reps each side

• **Don't forget your full body stretch!** •

TUESDAY • THURSDAY

- Head-to-Toe Stretches: 10 minutes total

- Your choice cardiovascular exercise (walk in place during the commercials or for 10 to 20 minutes continuously)

MEN'S WORKOUT

WORKOUT SCHEDULES

4

MONDAY • WEDNESDAY • FRIDAY

1st Commercial Break:

• Upper Body Stretches:	Neck	10 seconds
	Chest	10 seconds
	Shoulders	10 seconds
	Arms	10 seconds each arm
• Upper Body Exercises:	Pushups	5–7 reps
	Dips	5–7 reps
	Arm Kickbacks	8 reps each arm
	Arm Curls	8 reps each arm

2nd Commercial Break:

• Ab Stretch:	Stomach Stretch	15 seconds
	Lower Back	15 seconds
• Ab Exercises:	Four-Way Crunches	7–10 reps
	Oblique Situps	8 reps each side
	or Lovehandles	8 reps each side

3rd Commercial Break:

• Leg Stretches:	Toe Touch	10 seconds
	or Hurdler Stretch	10 seconds each leg
	Thigh Stretch	10 seconds each leg
	Calf Stretch	10 seconds each leg
• Leg Exercises:	Squats	7–10 reps
	Lunges	5–7 reps each leg
	Heel Raises	10 reps each leg

4th Commercial Break:

• Ab Stretch:	Stomach Stretch	15 seconds
• Stomach Exercises:	Four-Way Crunches	7–10 reps
	Oblique Situps	7–10 reps each side

• **Don't forget your full body stretch!** •

TUESDAY • THURSDAY

• Head-to-Toe Stretches: 10 minutes total

• Your choice cardiovascular exercise (walk in place during the commercials or for 10 to 20 minutes continuously)

MONDAY • WEDNESDAY • FRIDAY

 1st Commercial Break:

• Upper Body Stretches:	Neck	10 seconds
	Chest	10 seconds
	Shoulders	10 seconds
	Arms	10 seconds each arm
• Upper Body Exercises:	Pushups	6–9 reps
	Dips	6–9 reps
	Arm Kickbacks	9 reps each arm
	Arm Curls	9 reps each arm

 2nd Commercial Break:

• Ab Stretch:	Stomach Stretch	15 seconds
	Lower Back	15 seconds
• Ab Exercises:	Four-Way Crunches	8–11 reps
	Oblique Situps	9 reps each side
	or Lovehandles	9 reps each side

 3rd Commercial Break:

• Leg Stretches:	Toe Touch	10 seconds
	or Hurdler Stretch	10 seconds each leg
	Thigh Stretch	10 seconds each leg
	Calf Stretch	10 seconds each leg
• Leg Exercises:	Squats	8–11 reps
	Lunges	6–8 reps each leg
	Heel Raises	12 reps each leg

 4th Commercial Break:

• Ab Stretch:	Stomach Stretch	15 seconds
• Stomach Exercises:	Four-Way Crunches	8–11 reps
	Oblique Situps	8–11 reps each side

• Don't forget your full body stretch! •

TUESDAY • THURSDAY

• Head-to-Toe Stretches: 10 minutes total

• Your choice cardiovascular exercise (walk in place during the commercials or for 10 to 20 minutes continuously)

MONDAY • WEDNESDAY • FRIDAY

 1ST COMMERCIAL BREAK:

- Upper Body Stretches:
Neck	10 seconds
Chest	10 seconds
Shoulders	10 seconds
Arms	10 seconds each arm

- Upper Body Exercises:
Pushups	7–10 reps
Dips	7–10 reps
Arm Kickbacks	10 reps each arm
Arm Curls	10 reps each arm

 2ND COMMERCIAL BREAK:

- Ab Stretch:
Stomach Stretch	15 seconds
Lower Back	15 seconds

- Ab Exercises:
Four-Way Crunches	9–12 reps
Oblique Situps	10 reps each side
or Lovehandles	10 reps each side

 3RD COMMERCIAL BREAK:

- Leg Stretches:
Toe Touch	10 seconds
or Hurdler Stretch	10 seconds each leg
Thigh Stretch	10 seconds each leg
Calf Stretch	10 seconds each leg

- Leg Exercises:
Squats	9–12 reps
Lunges	14 reps each leg
Heel Raises	14 reps each leg

 4TH COMMERCIAL BREAK:

- Ab Stretch:
- Stomach Exercises:
Stomach Stretch	15 seconds
Four-Way Crunches	9–12 reps
Oblique Situps	9–12 reps each side

- **Don't forget your full body stretch!** •

TUESDAY • THURSDAY

- Head-to-Toe Stretches: 10 minutes total

- Your choice cardiovascular exercise (walk in place during the commercials or for 10 to 20 minutes continuously)

MEN'S WORKOUT

WORKOUT SCHEDULES

4

MONDAY • WEDNESDAY • FRIDAY

 1ST COMMERCIAL BREAK:

• Upper Body Stretches:	Neck	10 seconds
	Chest	10 seconds
	Shoulders	10 seconds
	Arms	10 seconds each arm
• Upper Body Exercises:	Pushups	8–11 reps
	Dips	8–11 reps
	Arm Kickbacks	11 reps each arm
	Arm Curls	11 reps each arm

 2ND COMMERCIAL BREAK:

• Ab Stretch:	Stomach Stretch	15 seconds
	Lower Back	15 seconds
• Ab Exercises:	Four-Way Crunches	10–13 reps
	Oblique Situps	11 reps each side
	or Lovehandles	11 reps each side

 3RD COMMERCIAL BREAK:

• Leg Stretches:	Toe Touch	10 seconds
	or Hurdler Stretch	10 seconds each leg
	Thigh Stretch	10 seconds each leg
	Calf Stretch	10 seconds each leg
• Leg Exercises:	Squats	10–13 reps
	Lunges	6–9 reps each leg
	Heel Raises	14 reps each leg

4TH COMMERCIAL BREAK:

• Ab Stretch:	Stomach Stretch	15 seconds
• Stomach Exercises:	Four-Way Crunches	10–13 reps
	Oblique Situps	10–13 reps each side

• Don't forget your full body stretch! •

TUESDAY • THURSDAY

• Head-to-Toe Stretches: 10 minutes total

• Your choice cardiovascular exercise (walk in place during the commercials or for 10 to 20 minutes continuously)

MEN'S WORKOUT

WORKOUT SCHEDULES

4

MONDAY • WEDNESDAY • FRIDAY

1ST COMMERCIAL BREAK:

• Upper Body Stretches:	Neck	10 seconds
	Chest	10 seconds
	Shoulders	10 seconds
	Arms	10 seconds each arm
• Upper Body Exercises:	Pushups	9–11 reps
	Dips	9–11 reps
	Arm Kickbacks	12 reps each arm
	Arm Curls	12 reps each arm

2ND COMMERCIAL BREAK:

• Ab Stretch:	Stomach Stretch	15 seconds
	Lower Back	15 seconds
• Ab Exercises:	Four-Way Crunches	11–13 reps
	Oblique Situps	12 reps each side
	or Lovehandles	12 reps each side

3RD COMMERCIAL BREAK:

• Leg Stretches:	Toe Touch	10 seconds
	or Hurdler Stretch	10 seconds each leg
	Thigh Stretch	10 seconds each leg
	Calf Stretch	10 seconds each leg
• Leg Exercises:	Squats	11–13 reps
	Lunges	7–9 reps each leg
	Heel Raises	16 reps each leg

4TH COMMERCIAL BREAK:

• Ab Stretch:	Stomach Stretch	15 seconds
• Stomach Exercises:	Four-Way Crunches	11–13 reps
	Oblique Situps	11–13 reps each side

• **Don't forget your full body stretch!** •

TUESDAY • THURSDAY

• Head-to-Toe Stretches: 10 minutes total

• Your choice cardiovascular exercise (walk in place during the commercials or for 10 to 20 minutes continuously)

MONDAY • WEDNESDAY • FRIDAY

1ST COMMERCIAL BREAK:

- Upper Body Stretches:

Neck	10 seconds
Chest	10 seconds
Shoulders	10 seconds
Arms	10 seconds each arm

- Upper Body Exercises:

Pushups	9–12 reps
Dips	9–12 reps
Arm Kickbacks	12 reps each arm
Arm Curls	12 reps each arm

2ND COMMERCIAL BREAK:

- Ab Stretch:

Stomach Stretch	15 seconds
Lower Back	15 seconds

- Ab Exercises:

Four-Way Crunches	11–14 reps
Oblique Situps	12 reps each side
or Lovehandles	12 reps each side

3RD COMMERCIAL BREAK:

- Leg Stretches:

Toe Touch	10 seconds
or Hurdler Stretch	10 seconds each leg
Thigh Stretch	10 seconds each leg
Calf Stretch	10 seconds each leg

- Leg Exercises:

Squats	11–14 reps
Lunges	7–10 reps each leg
Heel Raises	18 reps each leg

4TH COMMERCIAL BREAK:

- Ab Stretch:
- Stomach Exercises:

Stomach Stretch	15 seconds
Four-Way Crunches	11–14 reps
Oblique Situps	11–14 reps each side

- **Don't forget your full body stretch!** •

TUESDAY • THURSDAY

- Head-to-Toe Stretches: 10 minutes total

- Your choice cardiovascular exercise (walk in place during the commercials or for 10 to 20 minutes continuously)

LEVEL ① ② **❸**   WEEK **❶** ② ③ ④

MONDAY • WEDNESDAY • FRIDAY

1st Commercial Break:

• Upper Body Stretches:	Neck	10 seconds
	Chest	10 seconds
	Shoulders	10 seconds
	Arms	10 seconds each arm
• Upper Body Exercises:	Pushups	10–13 reps
	Dips	10–13 reps
	Arm Kickbacks	13 reps each arm
	Arm Curls	13 reps each arm

2nd Commercial Break:

• Ab Stretch:	Stomach Stretch	15 seconds
	Lower Back	15 seconds
• Ab Exercises:	Four-Way Crunches	12–15 reps
	Oblique Situps	13 reps each side
	or Lovehandles	13 reps each side

3rd Commercial Break:

• Leg Stretches:	Toe Touch	10 seconds
	or Hurdler Stretch	10 seconds each leg
	Thigh Stretch	10 seconds each leg
	Calf Stretch	10 seconds each leg
• Leg Exercises:	Squats	11–14 reps
	Lunges	8–11 reps each leg
	Heel Raises	18 reps each leg

4th Commercial Break:

• Ab Stretch:	Stomach Stretch	15 seconds
• Stomach Exercises:	Four-Way Crunches	12–15 reps
	Oblique Situps	12–15 reps each side

• **Don't forget your full body stretch!** •

TUESDAY • THURSDAY

• Head-to-Toe Stretches: 10 minutes total

• Your choice cardiovascular exercise (walk in place during the commercials or for 10 to 20 minutes continuously)

MONDAY • WEDNESDAY • FRIDAY

 1ST COMMERCIAL BREAK:

- Upper Body Stretches:
Neck	10 seconds
Chest	10 seconds
Shoulders	10 seconds
Arms	10 seconds each arm

- Upper Body Exercises:
Pushups	11–14 reps
Dips	11–14 reps
Arm Kickbacks	15 reps each arm
Arm Curls	15 reps each arm

 2ND COMMERCIAL BREAK:

- Ab Stretch:
Stomach Stretch	15 seconds
Lower Back	15 seconds

- Ab Exercises:
Four-Way Crunches	13–16 reps
Oblique Situps	15 reps each side
or Lovehandles	15 reps each side

 3RD COMMERCIAL BREAK:

- Leg Stretches:
Toe Touch	10 seconds
or Hurdler Stretch	10 seconds each leg
Thigh Stretch	10 seconds each leg
Calf Stretch	10 seconds each leg

- Leg Exercises:
Squats	13–16 reps
Lunges	10–13 reps each leg
Heel Raises	20 reps each leg

 4TH COMMERCIAL BREAK:

- Ab Stretch:
- Stomach Exercises:
Stomach Stretch	15 seconds
Four-Way Crunches	13–16 reps
Oblique Situps	13–16 reps each side

• Don't forget your full body stretch! •

TUESDAY • THURSDAY

- Head-to-Toe Stretches: 10 minutes total

- Your choice cardiovascular exercise (walk in place during the commercials or for 10 to 20 minutes continuously)

MEN'S WORKOUT

WORKOUT SCHEDULES

4

MONDAY • WEDNESDAY • FRIDAY

 1ST COMMERCIAL BREAK:

- Upper Body Stretches:
Neck	10 seconds
Chest	10 seconds
Shoulders	10 seconds
Arms	10 seconds each arm

- Upper Body Exercises:
Pushups	12–15 reps
Dips	12–15 reps
Arm Kickbacks	15 reps each arm
Arm Curls	15 reps each arm

 2ND COMMERCIAL BREAK:

- Ab Stretch:
Stomach Stretch	15 seconds
Lower Back	15 seconds
- Ab Exercises:
Four-Way Crunches	14–17 reps
Oblique Situps	15 reps each side
or Lovehandles	15 reps each side

 3RD COMMERCIAL BREAK:

- Leg Stretches:
Toe Touch	10 seconds
or Hurdler Stretch	10 seconds each leg
Thigh Stretch	10 seconds each leg
Calf Stretch	10 seconds each leg
- Leg Exercises:
Squats	14–17 reps
Lunges	10–13 reps each leg
Heel Raises	22 reps each leg

 4TH COMMERCIAL BREAK:

- Ab Stretch:
- Stomach Exercises:
Stomach Stretch	15 seconds
Four-Way Crunches	14–17 reps
Oblique Situps	14–17 reps each side

• **Don't forget your full body stretch!** •

TUESDAY • THURSDAY

- Head-to-Toe Stretches: 10 minutes total

- Your choice cardiovascular exercise (walk in place during the commercials or for 10 to 20 minutes continuously)

MONDAY • WEDNESDAY • FRIDAY

 ### 1st Commercial Break:

- Upper Body Stretches:
Neck	10 seconds
Chest	10 seconds
Shoulders	10 seconds
Arms	10 seconds each arm

- Upper Body Exercises:
Pushups	13–16 reps
Dips	13–16 reps
Arm Kickbacks	16 reps each arm
Arm Curls	16 reps each arm

 ### 2nd Commercial Break:

- Ab Stretch:
Stomach Stretch	15 seconds
Lower Back	15 seconds

- Ab Exercises:
Four-Way Crunches	15–18 reps
Oblique Situps	18 reps each side
or Lovehandles	18 reps each side

3rd Commercial Break:

- Leg Stretches:
Toe Touch	10 seconds
or Hurdler Stretch	10 seconds each leg
Thigh Stretch	10 seconds each leg
Calf Stretch	10 seconds each leg

- Leg Exercises:
Squats	15–18 reps
Lunges	11–14 reps each leg
Heel Raises	24 reps each leg

 ### 4th Commercial Break:

- Ab Stretch:
Stomach Stretch	15 seconds

- Stomach Exercises:
Four-Way Crunches	15–18 reps
Oblique Situps	15–18 reps each side

• Don't forget your full body stretch! •

TUESDAY • THURSDAY

- Head-to-Toe Stretches: 10 minutes total

- Your choice cardiovascular exercise (walk in place during the commercials or for 10 to 20 minutes continuously)

Dairy ——————

Meat ——————

Breads ——————

Vegetables ——————

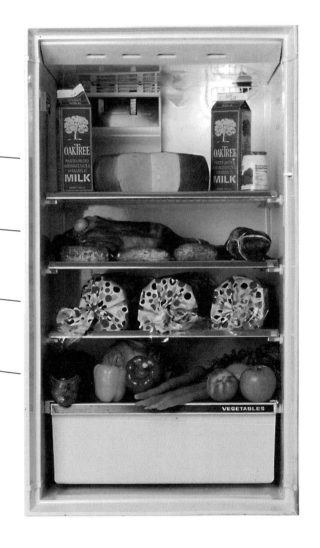

CHAPTER FIVE

Nutrition

Everyone wants to have more energy to do the things they enjoy. If you want to be energetic, you have to fill your body with the right fuel. Without the right fuel, your body will eventually break down, losing energy and the ability to fight off illness. It is very easy to avoid poor health, high doctor bills, and low self-esteem. All you have to do is *take care of yourself.*

This chapter is dedicated to teaching you how to take care of yourself. It will give you basic suggestions and advice on what foods to eat for more energy, how much to eat, and when to eat.

Water and Dehydration

Without question, one of the most important parts of your diet is the intake of water. To maintain a healthy and active lifestyle, water is an absolute necessity.

What do we know about the importance of water? You can live for weeks without food, but only for a few days without water. Almost two-thirds of your body is water. Your water percentage must remain that high in order to carry nutrients through the bloodstream to the organs and cells and to remove waste products. Your body uses water every day for breathing, perspiration, and excretion. Although most of us take it for granted, water may be the only true "cure" for permanent weight loss.

According to Donald S. Robertson, MD, MSC, who serves on the staff of the Scottsdale Memorial Hospital and is a frequent source of information for the FDA, water naturally suppresses the appetite and helps the body metabolize stored fat. Studies have shown that a decrease in water intake will cause fat deposits to increase, while an increase in water intake can actually reduce fat deposits.

Here is how water helps you lose weight. Your kidneys function best when your body is fully hydrated with water. When your kidneys aren't working at full capacity, some of their work load is dumped onto the liver. One of the liver's primary functions is to metabolize stored fat into usable energy for your body. But, if the liver has to do some of the kidney's work, it can't operate at full throttle either. As a result, your liver metabolizes less fat, more fat remains stored in your body, and weight loss stops.

Strange as it may seem, drinking enough water is also the best treatment for fluid retention. When the body gets less water, it will resort to what is commonly referred to as "camel mode" and begin to conserve every drop. That conserved water is stored in extra cellular spaces (outside the cells). This shows up as swollen feet, legs and hands. The best way to overcome the problem of water retention is to give your body what it needs— plenty of water. Only then will the retained water be released. Another reason you may have a constant problem with water retention is if you use too much salt on your food. Your body will tolerate sodium only in a certain concentration. The more salt you eat, the more water your system retains to dilute it. Luckily, getting rid of unneeded salt is easy—just drink more water! As water is forced through the kidneys, it takes away excess sodium.

Many people ask me, "How much water should I drink every day?" On the average, a person should drink eight 8-ounce glasses every day. If you exercise and perspire, you need to drink even more water, sometimes as much as ten 8-ounce glasses of water per day. I'd suggest that you have access to water all day and take a sip every few minutes. This will clean your system, give your body its daily requirement, and decrease your hunger at lunch and dinner.

However, the overweight person needs one additional glass of water for every 25 pounds of excess weight. That means, if you are 200 pounds overweight you should drink a gallon of water a day. This is because larger people have larger metabolic loads. Since we know that water is the key to fat metabolism, it makes sense that the overweight person needs more water.

Many people think they need to sweat to lose weight. This is not true! In fact, sweating is nothing more than the body cooling itself. The water lost to sweating must be replaced as soon as possible, or you will run the risk of dehydration. Your body can only handle about a four to five percent loss of fluid. Once you reach that level, you will feel sick, tired, and have a headache. It's obvious that water consumption is extremely important to good health.

Some Common Facts About Drinking Water

- Drinking water is essential to weight loss.
- To get rid of excess water weight, you must drink more water.
- The body can't metabolize stored fat efficiently without being fully hydrated.
- Retained water could be a majority of your excess weight.
- When you drink water, more fat is used as fuel because the liver is free to metabolize stored fat. Thus you will lose more weight.

Caffeine, Nicotine, and Alcohol

Caffeine, nicotine, and alcohol all absorb the water in our bodies. You must be careful when you use products that contain these substances, and try to drink at least one cup of water after you drink a cup of coffee or soda, smoke a cigarette, or have an alcoholic beverage. Of the three, alcohol is the worst absorber of water.

If you are a smoker or drinker of coffee or alcohol, try your best to curb these habits. Get help if you have to. These products will only make you less healthy as you age. If you choose not to quit (which is your prerogative), once again, drink water every time you smoke a cigarette or drink caffeinated or alcoholic beverages.

If you drink alcohol, you should limit your daily intake to no more than 1 to 2 drinks. There are numerous reasons to limit your consumption of alcohol. First, there is a strong link between alcohol use and malnutrition, anemia, high blood pressure and cancer. Second, like sugar, alcohol contains empty calories. These empty calories are stored in the fatty tissue around your legs, buttocks and waist.

After researching studies by the National Institute of Health and the U.S. Surgeon General, I was shocked to learn that over 50 million Americans smoke tobacco. As you learned in the earlier chapters, 97 million Americans are overweight and need to begin an exercise program. So, if you add two and two together, you might deduce that an estimated 30–40% of the 97 million target audience of this workout program smoke tobacco. It seems safe to say that most smokers are not exercisers or health-conscious.

NUTRITION

5

Quitting smoking has significant benefits at any age. Quitting decreases the risk of lung and other cancers, heart attack, stroke and chronic disease. Physically, your blood pressure and heart rate can decrease, meaning that your circulatory system is working more efficiently. Although a majority of smokers want to quit smoking, attempts to do so often fail. Yet quitting is very possible; in fact, the majority of people who smoke do give up cigarettes eventually, though only 20% are successful on their first attempt. Most people will give up several times before finally stopping for good.

The good news for quitters is that they will achieve the same health levels as nonsmokers after a few years, especially if they stop while they are young. Even older lifetime smokers can benefit significantly from quitting. Yes, the human body is an amazing life force —it will repair itself *if* you let it.

If you smoke you know there is no simple remedy for quitting. It helps to find a personal reason, instead of responding to relatives' or friends' complaints. Most quitters stop on their own —sometimes with the help of books, pamphlets, guides, or videos. Some prefer group support or professional counseling from a doctor or a smoking clinic. No single method works for everyone, so you may have to experiment with several of the above methods if you are seriously contemplating quitting. Keep in mind, though, that the withdrawal symptoms subside more quickly for smokers who quit all at once than for those who gradually cut down.

Good News About Weight Gain After Quitting

 Many smokers do not want to quit for fear of gaining weight if they stop smoking. Studies show that many of those who quit do gain weight, but the gain is usually only a few pounds, and can be minimized by exercising and eating low-fat foods and drinking more water.

Food and Your Eating Habits

You bought this exercise program because you thought you needed to be healthier. To achieve the level of healthiness you desire, the only adjustments you need to make are easy: exercise a little more and eat a little less during the evenings and in between meals. As well, you'll have to watch the level of fat in your diet, and avoid foods high in fat. A balanced diet, and eating in moderation—these two concepts will help you maintain a healthier lifestyle. It isn't too tough to do, if you have a guideline to follow.

If you ask people to name the four food groups, many would not be able to answer you confidently. Here is a chart of the four food groups and servings you need per day of each (Fruits and vegetables constitute one food group, but your diet should include servings of each per day):

3 =3

Food Group	Servings		
	1,600 Calories	2,200 Calories	2,800 Calories
Breads	6	9	11
Vegetables	3	4	5
Fruits	2	3	4
Dairy products	2	2	2
Meats (ounces)	5	6	7

Source: Modified from the U.S. Department of Agriculture, The Food Guide Pyramid (Home and Garden Bulletin No. 252), Washington, D.C.: USDA, 1992.

The chart is based on a 1,600-calorie, 2,200-calorie, and 2,800-calorie diet. Your calorie intake will vary depending on the amount of weight you want to lose, your body type and weight, and your age. If you eat from this list you cannot go wrong!

The biggest change in your diet will be in making breakfast the biggest and most important meal of the day. Breakfast should be the meal with the most calories as well as the most nutritious in order to successfully conquer your schedule for the day. You should follow this saying, "Eat like a king at breakfast, a prince at lunch, and a pauper at dinner." Here are some ideas for breakfast, lunch, and dinner.

Food Group	Serving Size
Breads	1 slice of bread 1 ounce of ready-to-eat cereal ½ cup of cooked cereal, rice, or pasta
Vegetables	1 cup of raw leafy vegetables ½ cup of other vegetables, cooked or chopped raw ¾ cup of vegetable juice
Fruits	1 medium apple, banana, or orange ½ cup of chopped, cooked, or canned fruit ¾ cup of fruit juice
Dairy products	1 cup of milk or yogurt 1½ ounces of natural cheese 2 ounces of process cheese
Meats	2 to 3 ounces of cooked lean meat, poultry, or fish ½ cup of cooked dry beans 1 egg 2 tablespoons of peanut butter

Source: U.S. Department of Agriculture, The Food Guide Pyramid (Home and Garden Bulletin No. 252), Washington, D.C.: USDA, 1992.

The Health Risks of a High-Fat Diet

There is a strong association between diet and developing degenerative diseases such as arteriosclerosis (a high build-up of fat in your arteries). If you eat high levels of saturated fat and cholesterol, such as are found in red meats and dairy products, fat may build up in your arteries. Eventually, the blood flow in your arteries will become restricted or completely blocked, causing a stroke or heart attack. However, certain foods rich in vitamin E (a natural antioxidant) can actually reduce your heart disease risk. These are:

- Fish
- Spinach
- Collard Greens
- Wheat germ

If you do not like these foods (and many people do not) a multivitamin with vitamin E will suffice.

A diet high in fats also seems to increase the risk of some cancers, although the exact reasons for this are unknown. Some authorities recommend a diet of less than 20 percent of calories from fat to reduce the risk of breast cancer.

Finding and Preparing the Right Foods

As with other types of dietary changes, the key word in reducing fat intake is moderation. Drastic changes in your diet are much more difficult to accept and maintain. In fact, a complete change in dietary habits is almost impossible and requires extraordinary discipline. Instead, balance your intake of low-fat foods and high-fat foods. Watch the portion size of protein-rich foods such as animal and dairy products. Eat more fruits, vegetables and grains. These foods are healthy, filling and low in fat, so make them the center of a meal, and use protein-rich foods for accent. So, instead of red meat and cheese, choose chicken or fish and plant proteins, such as peas and beans. Vegetable soup, whole-grain bread, and a salad, for instance, makes a great low-fat meal that is loaded with fiber, vitamins, and minerals.

Learn how to prepare your foods in a more healthy way too. Avoid frying chicken or fish. Grilling, broiling, and microwaving are good low-fat methods for cooking meats, poultry, and fish.

If you look at the Food Guide Pyramid, you'll notice that vegetables, fruits, and grains are the foundation of a healthy diet. It is absolutely necessary to eat more of these foods than any other food source. Fortunately, these foods are inexpensive and an excellent source of vitamins, minerals, and fiber. Vegetables, fruits, and grains are naturally low in fat and sodium and contain no cholesterol.

Sugar

Try to avoid foods high in sugar. These foods tend to have empty calories —calories without other nutrients. Besides adding calories, sugar is rapidly digested by the body and provides a quick energy source. If you do not use this quick energy source immediately your body will store the sugar as fat. Soda is one of the worst offenders of high-sugar content, and some Americans drink more than twelve cans of soda a day! The sugar in those sodas travels straight to your waist line, buttocks and hips.

Salt

Salt, or sodium, can increase blood pressure in susceptible people. Plus, we've already learned that too much sodium can cause weight gain due to water retention. Try to remember that there is really no need to use salt when cooking or eating. Use herbs and other spices to perk up a dish instead. Since many canned and processed foods are high in sodium, try to check labels before buying. The healthy daily maximum amount of sodium is about six grams.

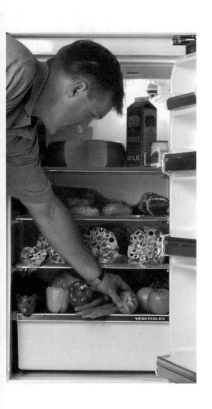

Eating Sensibly

Don't feel guilty if you decide to take a day off or have that urge to eat a dessert. Go ahead, and remember, "Everything in moderation." If you don't cheat on your workout and diet more than once a week, you'll be fine. Try to cheat only once a week or it will be difficult to get healthier and lose those extra pounds.

As you have probably already realized, this entire workout is designed so that you do not have to drastically change your lifestyle or eating habits. It is your decision to make a change in your life. You can do anything if you put your mind to it. So get started exercising, drop a few bad habits, and you're on your way to a healthy, happy life. Good luck!

Food Group	Eat These Foods Every Day	Eat These Foods Once a Week (Max) If At All
Fruits	Fresh / raw is best way to prepare: apples, oranges, bananas, grapes, peaches, tomatoes, pears, plums, raisins, juices of all (without sugar added)	Canned fruit (heavy syrup), fruit drinks, glazed fruit
Vegetables	Fresh / raw / steamed is the best way to prepare these: broccoli, green leafy lettuce, carrots, green beans, field peas, corn, cucumbers, squash	Canned vegetables (high in sodium), fried vegetables, french fries
Grains/Cereals/Nuts	Whole wheat breads, oatmeal, germ, pumpkin seeds (unsalted), whole wheat pasta (not refined), unsweetened cereal, baked potatoes, yams	White bread, refined pasta, white rice, prepared foods such as (pizza, macaroni and cheese, lasagna) sweet cereals, salted crackers, salted nuts, dinner rolls
Meat/Fish/Poultry	Fresh or frozen / trimmed fat tuna, crab, chicken, turkey (without the skin), lean meats	Commercial hamburger, hot dogs, cold cuts (prepared), poultry with skin, sausage, organ meats, ground beef, pork loin, fried chicken, bacon
Dairy Products	Milk, cheese, butter, oils, non-fat / skim milk, low-fat yogurt, margarine (made of corn, soy, sunflower oil), cottage cheese	Ice cream, whole milk, sour cream, butter, cooking with lard, eggs
Snacks / Desserts:	SENSITIVE SUBJECT TO SOME!! (REMEMBER MODERATION) (stay away from salty foods and the desire to eat sweets will be less) Cake, cookies, pies, ice cream, soda (huge amounts of sugar in soda) potato chips, salted / unsalted peanuts (high in fat)	
Also—Stay Away From:	Dressings for salads and vegetables, steak sauces, soy sauce, salt, meat gravy. Instead: Use natural herbs and spices for dressings and cooking, lemon juice on salads, pepper, tomato juices, onions	

The above was taken from the cupboards of the author. Yes, there are sodas, steaks, cookies, and chips in my cupboard as there are in most people's. Eating those foods rarely and in moderation is the key to not taking in too many calories each day. . . . Good Luck!—Stew Smith